Beyond Inherited: Personalized Medicine

Nina

First Printing, 2024

Contents

Chapter 1: Introduction

1.1 Overview

Whole genome/exome sequencing (WGS/WES) has been developed to study genetic variations, especially effective in detecting mutation associated to genetic disorders. The experiments often collected samples in a trio design so mutations only present in child patients but not in parents can be identified and further studied on implicated risk genes. Those mutations are commonly called as "*de novo*" mutations. Studies on developmental disorders heavily impacted by genetic risk factors found that *de novo* Loss-of-function (LoF) mutations are indeed significant genetic contributions to diseases, such as autism spectrum disorder (ASD) (Iossifov et al., 2014) and congenital heart disease (CHD) (Jin et al., 2017). A WES study on *de novo* mutations in autism identified significant contribution from *de novo* likely-gene disrupting mutaitons (LGDs), or commonly called as LoF mutations (Figure 1.1). The enrichment rate of

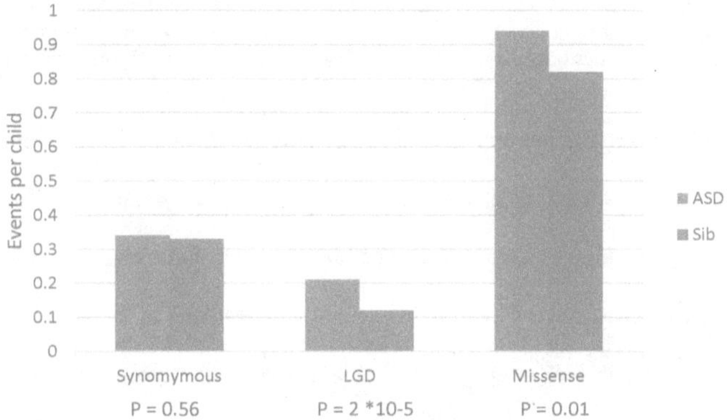

Figure 1.1 De novo variants comparison between affected patients and unaffected siblings. The event counts for likely-gene disrupting mutations (LGDs) are in the largest discrepancy between cases (ASD) and controls (Sib), indicating the contribution of *de novo* LGD mutations to autism. The figure is adapted from Iossifov et al., 2014.

LGDs comparing cases and controls is 1.75 (0.21/0.12), which means about 43% LGDs are pathogenic variants. While the enrichment rate for missense variants is 1.15 (0.94/0.82), indicating only 13% *de novo* missense variants are pathogenic. However, current statistic power has not been sufficient to distinguish the risk variants from the random ones because of limited recurrency of those variants (Figure 1.2). A previous study on de novo LGD mutations from CHD showed that only a small proportion of LGD variants located in the same gene which is the

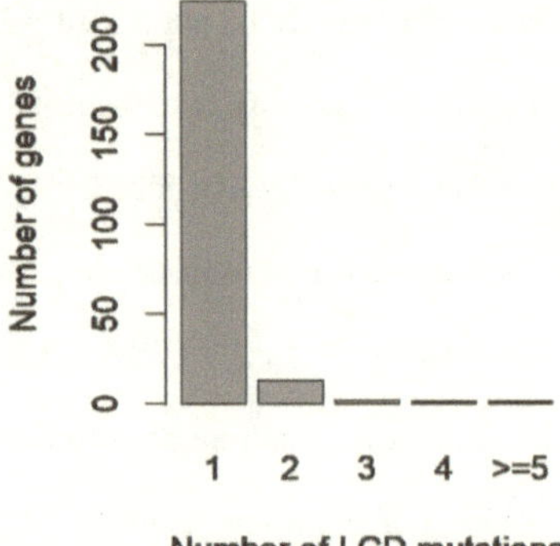

Figure 1.2 Risk gene discovery by recurrence is limited. The number of de novo LGD variants contained in each gene shows that only a small proportion of risk genes have recurrent mutations. Most risk variants only occur once, which makes it harder to identify. The figure is adapted from Jin et al., 2017.

great hurdle to identify risk genes and study disease etiology (Jin et al., 2017). I am going to review in section 1.2 on some typical statistic methods developed for risk gene discovery.

The work in this thesis took a different perspective from functional genomic data to identify disease risk genes rather than utilizing genomic data solely. In the meantime, by integrating functional data such as epigenome or single-cell transcriptome, we can impart vulnerable cell types or developmental stages specific to a disease altogether. In section 1.3, gene dosage sensitivity is reviewed and the most implicated disease mechanism by genetic variants, haploinsufficiency has also been illustrated. In the following sections 1.4 and 1.5, I reviewed how epigenomic modification regulates on transcription, what specific epigenomic patterns in haploinsufficient genes have and how important spatiotemporal expression is to development.

1.2 Statistical genetics for risk gene discovery by *de novo* variants

To better utilize WES data and reveal more disease risk genes, an integrated empirical Bayesian model, TADA (Transmission And *De novo* Association), has been developed to borrow information across all genes to infer parameters that would be difficult to estimate for individual genes. Based on a Hierarchical Bayesian framework, false discovery rate (FDR) for each gene can be calculated and the confidence for association between genes and a particular disease can be measure by FDR (X. He et al., 2013).

In TADA, two major parameters, relative risk of a gene causing a disease γ and the proportion of disease risk genes across whole genome π, are estimated by the connection to variant fold enrichment (***FE***), which is calculated as the number of observed variants divided by the number of expected. Assuming the background mutation rate for each gene is μ, total number of genes in the genome is m and total number of sequenced samples is N, then

the observed variants, $X = \pi m \times 2\gamma\mu N + (1-\pi)m \times 2\mu N$

the expected variants, $X_e = \pi m \times 2\mu N + (1-\pi)m \times 2\mu N$

$$FE = \frac{X}{Xe} = \pi(\gamma - 1) + 1,\ \gamma \sim Gamma\,(\bar{\gamma}\beta, \beta)$$

Since ***FE*** can be calculated from the data, β was fixed to 1 and estimate γ and π accordingly.

Bayes factor can be estimated as following:

$$B = \frac{P(X|H1)}{P(X|H0)} \sim \frac{Pois(2\gamma\mu N)}{Pois(2\mu N)}$$

$H1$ is alternative hypothesis and $H0$ is null, where $\gamma = 1$.

From Bayes' theorem, the posterior odds are equal to the Bayes factor times the prior odds:

$$\frac{P(H1|X)}{P(H0|X)} = \frac{P(X|H1)}{P(X|H0)} \times \frac{P(H1)}{P(H0)}$$

where $P(H1)$ is estimated π, $P(H0)$ is $(1-\pi)$.

Assuming $P(H1|X)$ is q, $P(H0|X)$ is $(1-q)$, the posterior probability of the null model is $q_0 = 1 - q$,

$$q = \frac{B\pi}{1-\pi+B\pi}$$

then per-gene based FDR can be calculated from q_0, which is the sum of total q_0 smaller than the current rank divided by the total number of genes with smaller q_0.

Another Bayesian method, extTADA developed based on the previous TADA and enabled estimation of parameters from local gene groups using Markov Chain Monte Carlo (MCMC) (Nguyen et al., 2017), which allow stratification of the genome based on prior knowledge and parameter estimation can be closer to the true story. We adapted this approach in our A-risk project discussed in Chapter 3, for identification of autism risk genes.

1.3 Gene dosage sensitivity

Dosage-sensitive genes are a subset of genes in our genome that can cause a phenotypic effect by a change in gene dosage, either in the way of duplication or deletion (Rice & McLysaght, 2017). There are 4 major mechanism of dosage sensitivity of a gene, haploinsufficiency, promiscuous off-target interactions at high concentration, dosage balance and concentration dependency (Figure 1.3). I am going to discuss each of them in the following.

Haploinsufficiency describes a phenomenon where a hemizygous state does not produce sufficient gene product for wildtype phenotypes, proposed by Wright as a source of dominant negative effects(S. Wright, 1934). This is the most intuitive form of dosage sensitivity, which is also the main etiology of *de novo* loss-of-function (LoF) variants identified through whole exome sequencing (WES) and whole genome sequencing (WGS) since most of the variants occur in one allele due to extremely low frequency. One well-studied example of haploinsufficiency is the 22q11 deletion syndrome, causing serious neural abnormalities such as schizophrenia or schizoaffective disorders (Karayiorgou, Simon, & Gogos, 2010). A study on protein-coding variation in 60,706 humans measured the depletion of LoF mutations in this relatively healthy population and grouped the constraint genes by how much less the observed LoF variants compared to the expected (Lek et al., 2016). They defined haploinsufficient genes by that the number of observed LoF variants within the gene is less than 10% of the expected and they derived a pLI score measuring haploinsufficiency with about 3000 genes in pLI >= 0.9.

By contrast, the presence of a surplus copy of a wild-type gene can also be deleterious (Figure 1.3b). For example, extra copies of the alpha-synuclein gene (*SNCA*) are associated with early-onset Parkinson's disease, possibly owing to greater protein concentration increasing the likelihood of protein aggregation and further precipitating as insoluble amyloid fibrils (Irvine, El-Agnaf, Shankar, & Walsh, 2008).

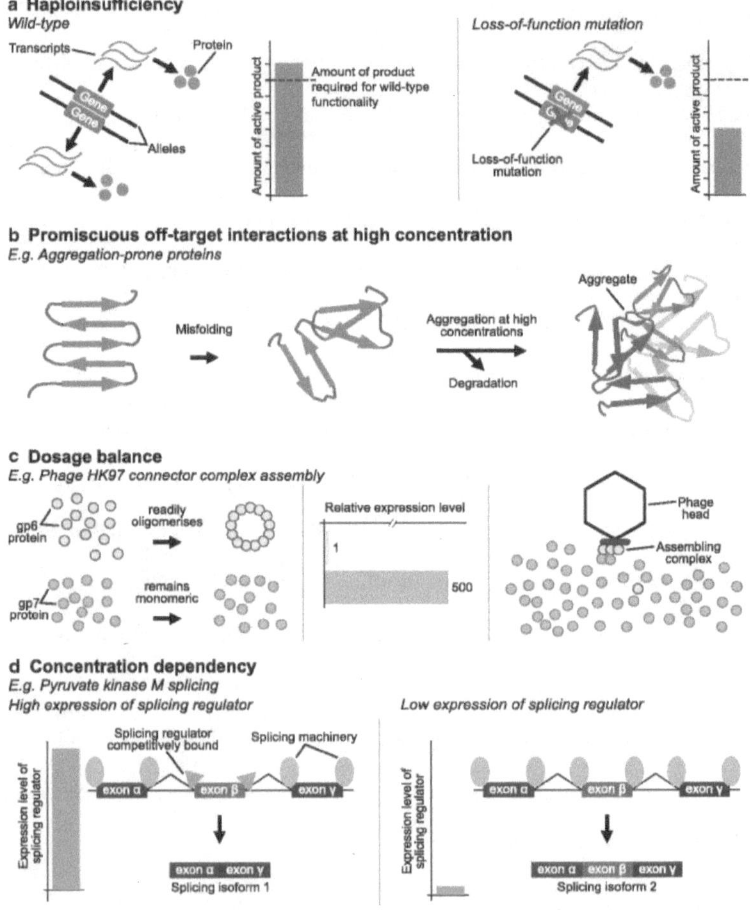

Figure 1.3 A general introduction to gene dosage sensitivity. There are 4 main types of dosage sensitivity functional through different mechanisms. Adapted from Rice&McLysaght, 2017.

On the other hand, some genes are sensitive to both situation and functioning within a concentration balance, which means they cause phenotypes when the copy number either increases or decreases. Protein components of large complexes can be particularly dosage-balanced because incorrect ratios of subunits can devastate the biochemistry of the complex assembly, leading to a disfunction of the protein complex. Sometimes a large increase of a subunit can result in a decrease in productions of the protein complex, such as the phage HK97 connector complex assembly (Cardarelli, Maxwell, & Davidson, 2011).

While the concentration balance can sometimes become an indicator for gene functions. For example, the pyruvate kinase M (PKM) is present in two isoforms during embryonic or adult stages. The spliced isoform is dependent on the concentration of hnRNP (heterogeneous nuclear ribonucleoproteins) proteins, where the concentration of the splicing regulator determines its location of binding and further determines which isoform is produced. A deleterious case is found in cancer cells with high concentrations of hnRNP proteins leading to the ectopic production of embryonic form (M. Chen, David, & Manley, 2012).

The study described in Chapter 2 mainly focused on characterization of disease risk genes less tolerant to heterozygous mutations, in other words haploinsufficient genes. We found specific connections between transcriptional regulation of haploinsufficient genes and epigenomic modification, based on which we further predict on additional haploinsufficient genes that have been understudied. Discovery on risk genes implicated in other dosage sensitivity mechanism is very important, but will definitely require more complicated models, which will not be the main topic of the thesis.

1.4 Epigenomic regulation

Epigenomic markers and features have been profiled and studied widely because of technical development. They can be generally grouped into six categories: 1. DNA level modifications usually occurring at position C5 or N3 on cytosines and N6 on adenines; 2. Histone level modifications occurring at more than 130 post-transcriptional modification (PTM) sites at the tails of the four core histones (H2A, H2B, H3 and H4); 3. The structurally different features such as nucleosome occupancy; 4. The chromatin interactions based on enhancers, promotors or insulators interactions; 5. The chromatin domain features profiled by Hi-C allowing studies on segmentation of the epigenome; 6. Non-coding RNA modifications regulating gene expression (Stricker, Koferle, & Beck, 2017). Among the six categories, histone level modifications have been the most well-studied (Figure 1.4). Active promotors are commonly demarcated by histone H3 lysine 4 dimethylation (H3K4me2), H3K4me3, acetylation (ac) and H2A.Z. Transcribed regions are enriched with H3K36me3 and H3K79me2. Repressed genes

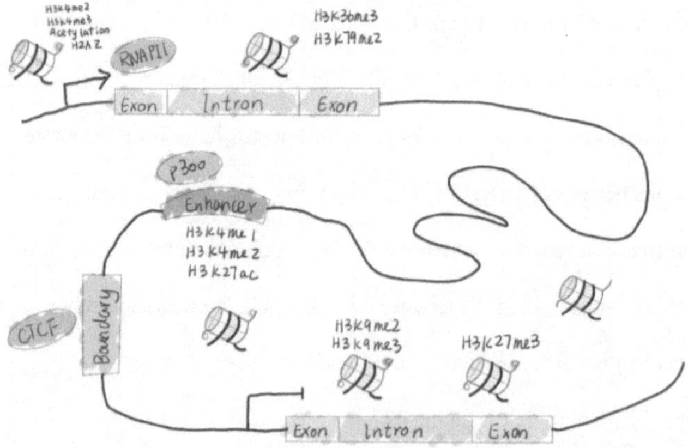

Figure 1.4 Histone modifications and their functions in genomic and transcriptomic regulation. Different histone modifications located in various functional genomic regions and distinguished functional elements. The figure is adapted from Zhou, Goren, & Bernstein, 2011.

may locate within large domains of H3K9me2 or H3K9me3 or H3K27me3. H3K4me1, H3K4me2, H3K27ac and the histone acetyltransferase p300 are usually enriched in enhancers. CCCTC-binding factors (CTCFs) bind to sites that function as boundary elements, insulators or structural scaffolds (Zhou, Goren, & Bernstein, 2011).

Histone modifications play an important role in sculping cell-type specific transcription. A recent study conducted a proximity ligation-assisted chromatin immunoprecipitation sequencing (PLAC-seq) (Fang et al., 2016) to identify chromatin interactions at active promoters marked by H3K4me3 in several major neuronal cell types, such as radial glia (RG), intermediate progenitor cells (IPCs), excitatory neurons (eNs) and interneurons (iNs) (Song et al., 2020). They mapped some key lineage-specific transcription factors' binding motif to the detected interaction regions and found that the motif enrichment aligned in accordance with the role of transcription factors in cell-type developmental trajectory. For example, the motifs for DLX1, DLX2, DLX6, GSX2 and LHX6 are enriched in interneurons, reflecting their roles in maturation and function of interneurons. The broad domains of H3K4me3 markers has also been identified association to transcriptional consistency, revealing interplays between histone modifications and transcriptional regulation. A previous study measured transcriptional consistency (lower transcriptional variability, or "transcriptional noise") in single cells by calculating the variance in expression relative to expression level for each gene in single-cell RNA-seq data sets (Benayoun et al., 2014). They found that genes marked by top 5% broadest H3K4me3 domains had reduced transcriptional variability across many different cell types, which indicates that H3K4me3 are critical for transcriptional precision by ensuring the robustness of transcriptional outputs.

Haploinsufficient genes are sensitive to expression level change, based on which derived a reasonable hypothesis that expression of haploinsufficient genes is under precise transcriptional regulation. A previous study analyzed thousands of genome-wide epigenetic profiles and found that tumor suppressor genes have broad H3K4me3 domains in normal cells (K. Chen et al., 2015a). Tumor suppressors are often implicated with germline risk in developmental disorders through haploinsufficiency (Qi, Dong, Chung, Wang, & Shen, 2016). Previous observations suggest that haploinsufficient genes may have specific pattern in epigenomic modifications in their functional genomic region, such as broader H3K4me3 peaks, to maintain a highly regulated and consistent transcriptomic expression.

1.5 Spatiotemporal gene expression

During the development of organisms, gene expression programs change over time, across differentiation and development, and in response to stimuli as well. A systematic study on mRNA microarray profiling of human prefrontal cortex collected the tissue from samples during a wide range of development, from fetus to late adulthood (Colantuoni et al., 2011). They measured the rate of expression changes in different developmental stages across the lifespan using a linear-spine model. The rate of expression change during fetal stages is much higher than at adulthood, even compared to the infant stage. However, after a steady platform throughout teenage years to the 40s, the rates rise again through several decades. This study vividly depicts the dynamics of gene expression on the time scale.

Cell-type specific gene expression is nowadays a critical topic in biological studies, especially when it comes to human diseases. For example, spatiotemporal expression of transcription factors (TFs) can precisely regulate organ development and physiology. A previous study on two homeobox transcription factors NKX2-5 and MEIS1 illustrates how spatiotemporal expression of TFs precisely regulates cardiogenesis (Dupays et al., 2015). NKX2-5 is also a haploinsufficient gene, mutations in which result in a spectrum of congenital heart disease of varying phenotypic penetrance (Akazawa & Komuro, 2005). During cardiac differentiation, the two transcription factors have partially overlapping expression patterns, with the result that as cardiac progenitors from the anterior heart field differentiate and migrate into the cardiac outflow tract, they sequentially experience high levels of MEIS1 and then increasing levels of NKX2-5 (Figure 1.5). The sequential binding provides a simple regulatory mechanism for a common pool of targets of these 2 TFs to regulate cardia development.

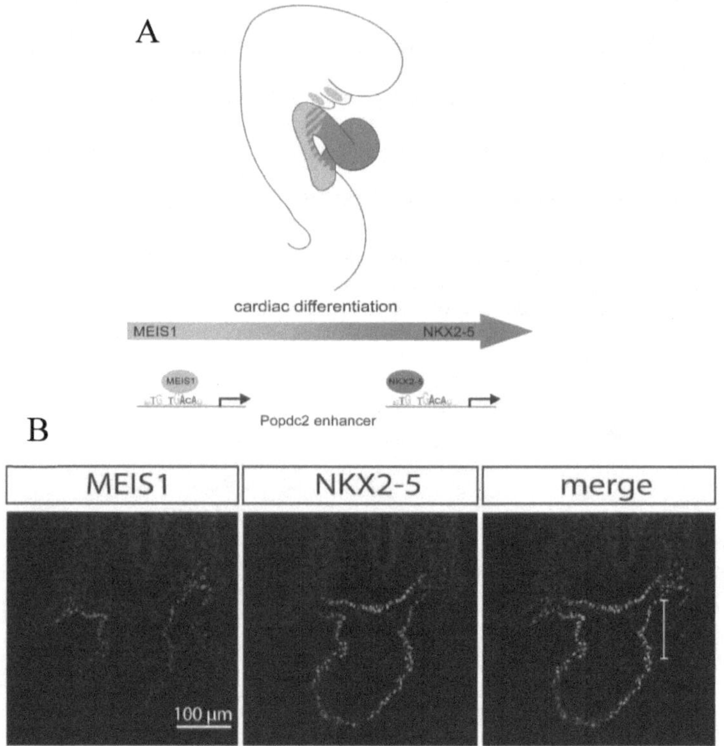

Figure 1.5 Spatial expression of two transcription factors NKX2-5 and MEIS1 in developing heart. (A) A graphic illustration of the distribution of two TFs expression. (B) Immunohistochemistry of NKX2-5 and MEIS1 on an E8.5 mouse embryo showing their colocalization in the distal outflow tract (OFT). The figures are adapted from Dupays et al., 2015.

With the development of Next-generation Sequencing (NGS) technology, people nowadays can capture a snapshot of gene expression or transcriptomic profiles in single cells.

Single-cell RNA sequencing is a powerful innovation that people can identify cell types with an unprecedented resolution in tissue heterogeneity (Klein & Treutlein, 2019) and gain insight on transcriptomic dynamic in a time scale of hours (La Manno et al., 2018). Besides, people can also study cell lineage construction with single-cell RNA-seq data, enabling better understanding of cellular differentiation and tissue development. Nowadays, there are in total of more than 500 single-cell transcriptomics studies available (Svensson, da Veiga Beltrame, & Pachter, 2019) (Figure 1.6). In the effort to better utilize so many data sets, large consortium projects have been launched to integrate them or generate single-cell data sets in a standard way. For example, The Human Cell Atlas portal aims to provide uniformly processed single-cell genomics data from all of the human body (Regev et al., 2017). Allen Brain Atlas collects functional genomic data of

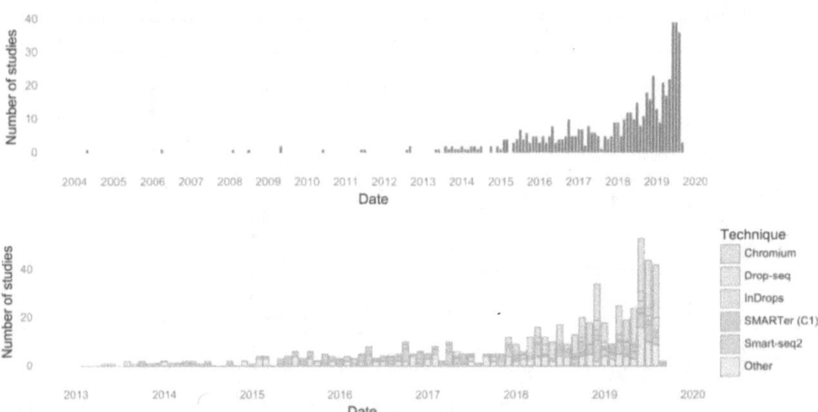

Figure 1.6 Single-cell transcriptomics studies over time. The lower panel stratified studies by different single-cell techniques. Single-cell studies are explosively increasing in recent years. The figures are adapted from Svensson, da Veiga Beltrame, & Pachter, 2019.

brains in human and mouse through a wide range of developmental stages to facilitate neuroscience studies (Miller et al., 2014).

Autism spectrum disorder (ASD) is a neurodevelopmental disorder mostly with very early onsets. With rapidly dynamic expression profiles in human fetal brain, we can hypothesize that autism risk genes affect specific neuronal cells or pathways during neuron differentiation and development. Gene expression level may provide a molecular basis for the pathogenic effect of dosage-sensitive risk genes. Learning from autism risk genes' expression pattern in fetal brains not only helps us identify implicated cell types and disease etiology, but also discover novel genetic risk in autism. In Chapter 3, we will discuss in detail how we use single-cell expression patterns of known autism risk genes to predict novel risk genes and infer affected neuronal cell types or brain structures.

Chapter 2: Distinct Epigenomic Patterns Are Associated with Haploinsufficiency and Predict Risk Genes of Developmental Disorders

2.1 Introduction

Haploinsufficiency (HIS) due to hemizygous deletions or heterozygous likely-gene-disrupting (LGD) variants plays a central role in the pathogenesis of various diseases. Recent large-scale exome and genome sequencing studies of developmental disorders, including autism, intellectual disability, developmental delay, and congenital heart disease (De Rubeis et al., 2014; Deciphering Developmental Disorders, 2015; Hamdan et al., 2014; Jason Homsy et al., 2015; Iossifov et al., 2014), have estimated that *de novo* LGD mutations explain the cause of a significant portion of patients with these developmental disorders, and the enrichment rate of *de novo* LGD variants indicates about half of these variants are associated with disease risk. However, relatively few genes have multiple LGD variants ("recurrence") in a cohort (De Rubeis et al.; Iossifov et al.; McRae et al.), lacking of which provides insufficient statistical evidence to distinguish individual risk genes from the ones with random mutations (X. He et al.). On the other hand, most of the enrichment of LGD variants can be explained by HIS genes (McRae et al.). Therefore, a comprehensive catalog of HIS genes can greatly help interpreting and prioritizing mutations in genetic studies.

Currently, there are two main approaches of predicting HIS genes based on high-throughput data. Huang et al. uses a combination of genetic, transcriptional and protein-protein interaction features from various sources to estimate haploinsufficient probabilities for 12,443 genes (Huang, Lee, Marcotte, & Hurles, 2010). Using similar input information, Steinberg et al. generated the probabilities for more (over 19,700) human genes by a Support Vector Machine (SVM) model (Steinberg, Honti, Meader, & Webber, 2015). The other approach is based on mutation intolerance (Cassa et al.; Lek et al., 2016; Petrovski, Wang, Heinzen, Allen, & Goldstein, 2013) in populations that do not have early onset developmental disorders. Lek et al

2016 (Lek et al.) estimated each gene's probability of haploinsufficiency (pLI: Probability of being Loss-of-function Intolerant) based on the depletion of rare LGD variants in over 60,000 exome sequencing samples. Although effective, ExAC pLI is biased towards genes with longer transcripts or higher background mutation rates, since the statistical power of assessing the significance depends on a relatively large expected number of rare LGD variants from background mutations.

We sought to predict HIS using epigenomic data that are orthogonal to genetic variants and generally independent of gene size. Our method is motivated by recent studies indicating that specific epigenomic patterns are associated with genes that are likely haploinsufficient. Specifically, genes with increased breadth of H3K4me3, typically associated with actively transcribing promoters, are enriched with tumor suppressor genes (K. Chen et al., 2015b), which are predominantly haploinsufficient based on somatic mutation patterns (Davoli et al., 2013). Another study reported H3K4me3 breadth regulates transcriptional precision (Benayoun et al., 2014), which is critical for dosage sensitivity. These observations led us to hypothesize that haploinsufficient genes are tightly regulated by a combination of transcription factors and epigenomic modifications to achieve spatiotemporal precision of gene expression, and such regulation can be detected by distinct patterns of epigenomic marks in relevant tissues and cell types. Based on this model, we developed a Random Forest–based method ("Episcore") using epigenomic data from the Epigenomic Roadmap (Roadmap Epigenomics et al., 2015) and ENCODE Projects (Consortium et al., 2012) as input features and a few hundreds of curated HIS genes as positive training data. To assess the performance of prioritizing candidate risk variants in real-world genetic studies, we used large data sets of *de novo* mutations from recent studies of birth defects and neurodevelopmental disorders and showed that Episcore had better performance than existing methods. Additionally, Episcore is less biased by gene length or background mutation rate and complementary to mutation-based metrics in HIS-based gene prioritization. Our analysis indicates that epigenomic features in stem cells, brain tissues, and fetal tissues contribute more to Episcore than others.

2.2 Results

2.2.1 Haploinsufficient (HIS) and Haplosufficient (HS) genes show distinct distributions of epigenomic features

To examine the correlation of gene haploinsufficiency and epigenomic patterns, we analyzed ChIP-seq data from Roadmap and ENCODE projects, including active (H3K4me3, H3K9ac, and H2A.Z) and repressive (H3K27me3) promoter modifications, and marks associated with enhancers (H3K4me1, H3K27ac, DNase I hypersensitivity sites). We used the width of called ChIP-seq peaks for promoter features and counted the interacting number of promoters and enhancers within pre-defined topologically-associated domains (TADs) for enhancer features. As each histone modification is characterized in multiple cell types, we refer to the combination of an epigenomic modification and a cell type as one epigenomic feature. Figure 2.1A shows the correlation among epigenomic features, and the correlation of epigenomic features and ExAC pLI score. As expected, active promoter or enhancer marks are highly correlated with each other and with ExAC pLI score, and they are anti-correlated with repressor marks in general. The repressor marks from stem cells or fetal tissues have positive correlations with active marks and ExAC pLI scores, suggesting many genes with bivalent marks in stem cells are likely haploinsufficient.

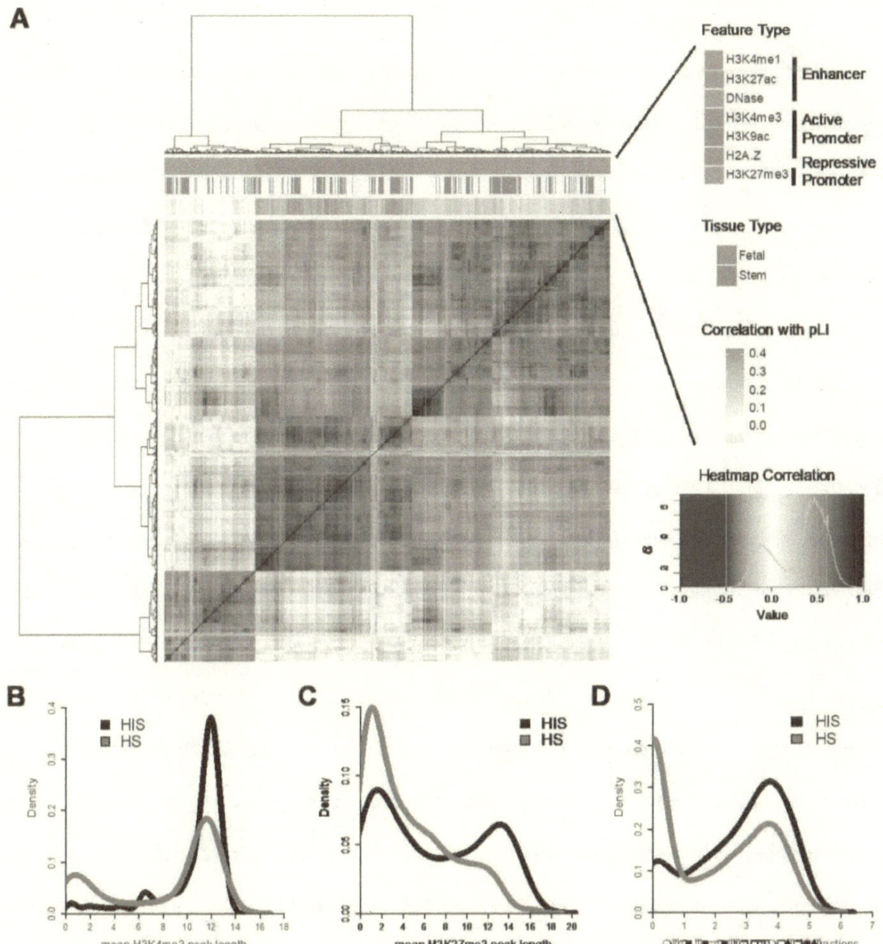

Figure 2.1 Epigenomic profiles are associated with gene haploinsufficiency. (A) Heatmap showing Spearman correlation between epigenomic features. Three groups of epigenomic features are included: active promoter, repressive promoter and enhancer features. Epigenomic features inside each group strongly correlate with each other. Different feature types, including various histone modifications, histone variant, and DNase I hypersensitivity sites, are color-coded. Above the heatmap, a bar denoting Spearman correction between epigenomic features and pLI shows many epigenomic features relate to HIS with varying degree. Data from stem cells or fetal tissues are also marked by color lines. (B-C) Known HIS and HS genes have different distributions of peak length of promoter features (B, H3K4me3; C, H3K27me3). For each gene, peak length was averaged across tissues. (D) HIS and HS genes have different distributions of number of interacting enhancers inferred by Epitensor. For each gene, the number of interacting enhancers was averaged across tissues.

To further investigate the association of haploinsufficiency and patterns of epigenomic modifications, we compiled a list of 287 known HIS genes (Supplementary Table 2.1) involved in a wide range of human diseases (Supplementary Table 2.2) from a recent study (Dang, Kassahn, Marcos, & Ragan, 2008; Huang et al., 2010) and human-curated ClinGen dosage sensitivity map. We also collected a list of 717 HS genes, of which one copy of each gene had been deleted in two or more subjects based on a CNV study in 2,026 healthy individuals (Shaikh et al., 2009). For promoter features, HIS and HS genes clearly have distinct distributions of peak length (Figure 2.1B-D). HIS genes on average have wider peaks of both the active marker H3K4me3 (Figure 2.1B) and the repressive marker H3K27me3 (Figure 2.1C), suggesting the difference between HIS and HS genes is not only on the level of expression but also on distinct mechanisms of regulation. Furthermore, other epigenomic modifications associated with active promoters, including H2A.Z and H3K9ac, also display wider peaks upstream of HIS genes (Figure 2.2 A and B). In addition, HIS and HS genes also differ in the number of interacting enhancers. We adopted a recently published method *EpiTensor* (Zhu et al., 2016), which decomposes a 3D tensor representation of histone modifications, DNase-Seq, and RNA-Seq data to find associations between distant genomic regions. When restricted to pre-defined topologically-associated domains (TADs), associated regions identified by *EpiTensor* correspond well to enhancer-promoter interactions found by Hi-C[20]. *EpiTensor* revealed that HIS genes have a median of 9 interacting enhancers, while HS genes have a median of 0 ($p < 10^{-4}$, permutation test, Figure 2.2C). When averaged across tissues, HIS genes shift towards a larger number of mean interacting enhancers, as compared to HS genes (Figure 2.1D), supporting the notion that HIS genes have more regulatory complexity.

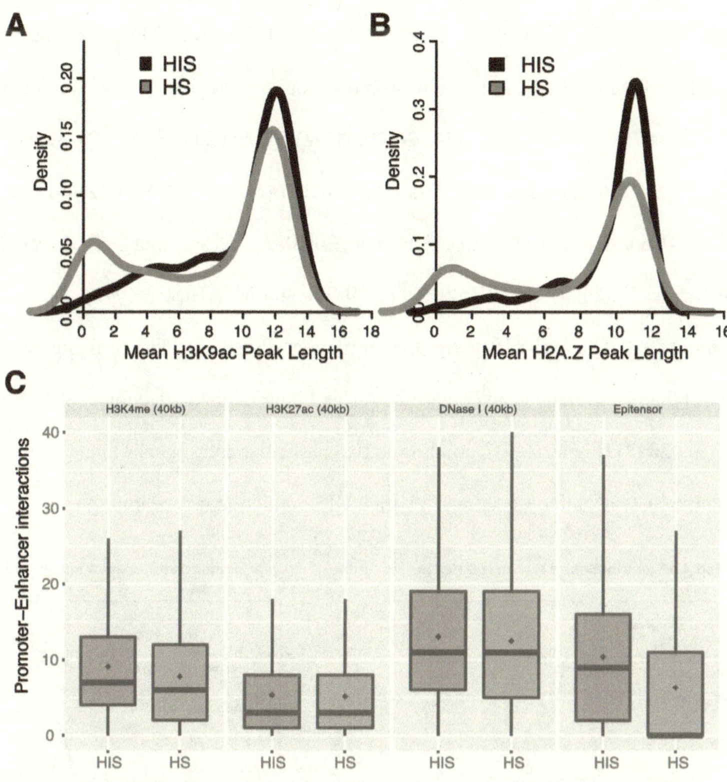

Figure 2.2 The disparity of HIS and HS genes in the distribution of epigenetic features. (A-B) HIS and HS genes have different distributions of peak length from promoter features (A, H3K9ac; B, H2A.Z). (C) HIS genes have larger numbers of interacting enhancers than HS genes. When interacting enhancers were measured as the number of peaks in +/- 20kb of TSS (C, the left 3 panels), little difference between HIS and HS genes were observed. When interacting enhancers were inferred by EpiTensor (C, the rightmost panel), there is significant difference between HIS and HS genes (p < 10-4, permutation test of difference between medians).

Among these 287 known HIS genes, 129 genes (45%) have pLI smaller than 0.9 or missing value. Some of these genes are well-known disease risk genes under dominant genetic models, such as *TGFB1*(Kinoshita et al., 2000), *RUNX1*(Taketani et al., 2002), *SOX2*(Fantes et al., 2003), *SUMO1*(Alkuraya et al., 2006), *NKX2-5*(Benson et al., 1999), *EYA4*(Wayne et al., 2001), *CAV1*(Cao, Alston, Ruschman, & Hegele, 2008), *PAX2*(Sanyanusin et al., 1995), *GATA6*(Kodo et al., 2009), *ZIC2*(Brown et al., 1998), and *WT1*(Hastie, 1992). These known HIS genes with pLI < 0.9 have significantly smaller number of expected loss of function variants(Lek et al., 2016) than an average gene (Figure 2.3A), and intermediate selection coefficient (S_{het}) (Cassa et al., 2017) (Figure 2.3B), pointing to two particular areas (genes that are either short or under intermediate negative selection) in which HIS prediction can be improved.

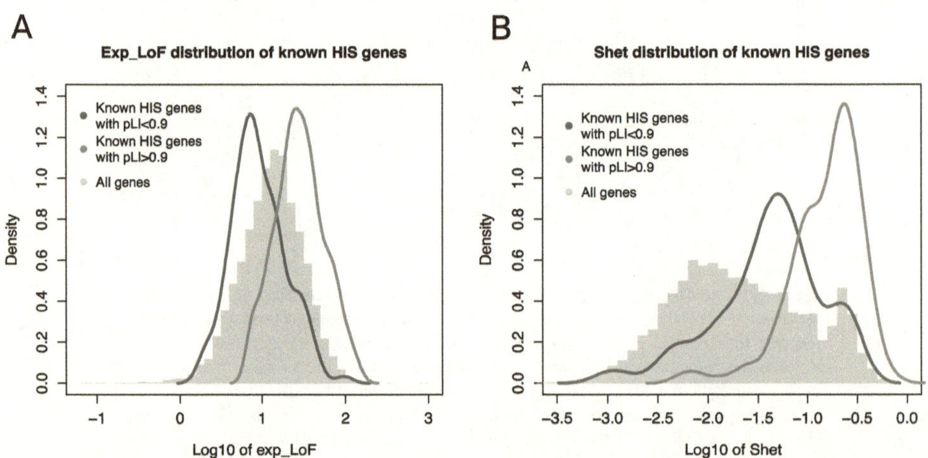

Figure 2.3 Property of mutation intolerance and selection of known haploinsufficient genes used in training. The known genes are divided into two groups based on ExAC pLI scores: above (red) and below (blue) 0.9. (A) The number of expected loss of function (exp_LoF)(Lek et al., 2016) distribution of genes with pLI >0.9 or pLI<0.9. The exp_LoF value is proportional to background mutation rate, which in turn is largely determined by transcript size. Known HIS genes with pLI < 0.9 have significantly smaller exp_LoF than an average gene, and the ones with pLI > 0.9 have much larger exp_LoF. (B) The S_{het} (average select coefficient of heterozygous loss of function variants in a gene) distribution of genes with pLI>0.9 or pLI<0.9. S_{het} values. Known HIS genes with pLI < 0.9 have intermediate S_{het}: larger than than an average gene but smaller than the ones with pLI > 0.9.

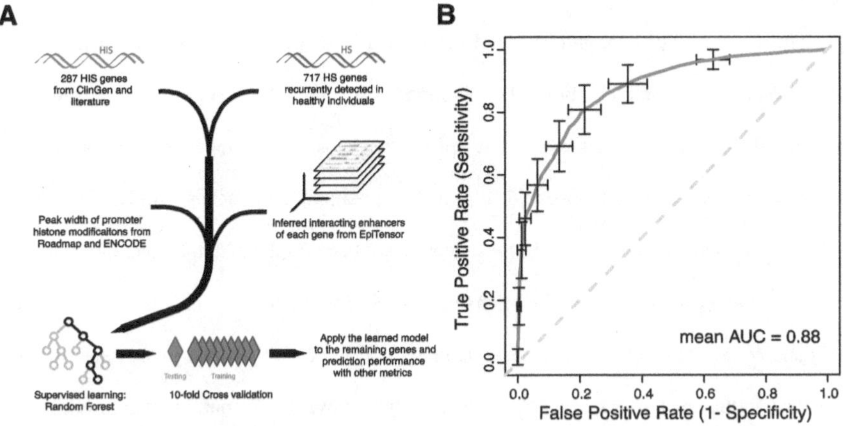

Figure 2.4 A Random Forest model to predict haploinsufficiency. (A) A flowchart of the method. (B) ROC curve from 10-fold cross-validation. The red curve is the average of 100 randomized cross-validation runs, with error bar showing standard deviation. The mean and median AUC of the 100 runs are 0.88 and 0.89, respectively.

2.2.2 Predicting haploinsufficiency with epigenomic features

To leverage the strong association between epigenomic patterns and gene haploinsufficiency, we developed a computational method to predict haploinsufficiency using Random Forest (Figure 2.4A) and other supervised learning models (Figure 2.5 A and B). The input features included peak length of four promoter marks (H3K4me3, H3K9ac, H2A.Z and H3K27me3) and the number of EpiTensor-inferred interacting enhancers in various tissues. Performance evaluation by 10-fold cross validation and AUC (Area Under Curve) in ROC (Receiver Operating Characteristic) curves showed that all of these methods achieved high AUC values of 0.86~0.88 (Figure 2.4B and Figure 2.5 A and B). As Random Forest performs the best, results from Random Forest are chosen as final metrics measuring the probability of being haploinsufficient, termed “Episcore” (Supplementary Table 2.3). Despite completely different input data are used, Episcore and ExAC pLI score displayed overall concordance. The distribution of pLI is generally bi-modal, with modes at 1 and 0 (Lek et al.). The genes with Episocre >0.6 are much more likely to have pLI values close to 1 than genes with Episocre < 0.4, and the opposite trend at pLI close to 0 (Figure 2.5C). Among 3463 genes with Episcore > 0.6, 1518 have pLI scores < 0.5. Some of these genes have been implicated in human diseases under a dominant model, such as *HEY2*(Reamon-Buettner & Borlak, 2006), *ASF1A*(Giannakou et al., 2017) and *HAND2*(Sun et al., 2016) (Supplementary Table 2.4). Similarly to the ones with low pLI values in the positive training set, these genes have lower background mutation rate (which is primarily determined by transcript size) than the ones with large pLI values (Figure 2.5D), and are generally under less severe selection measured by S_{het} (Cassa et al., 2017) (Figure 2.5E).

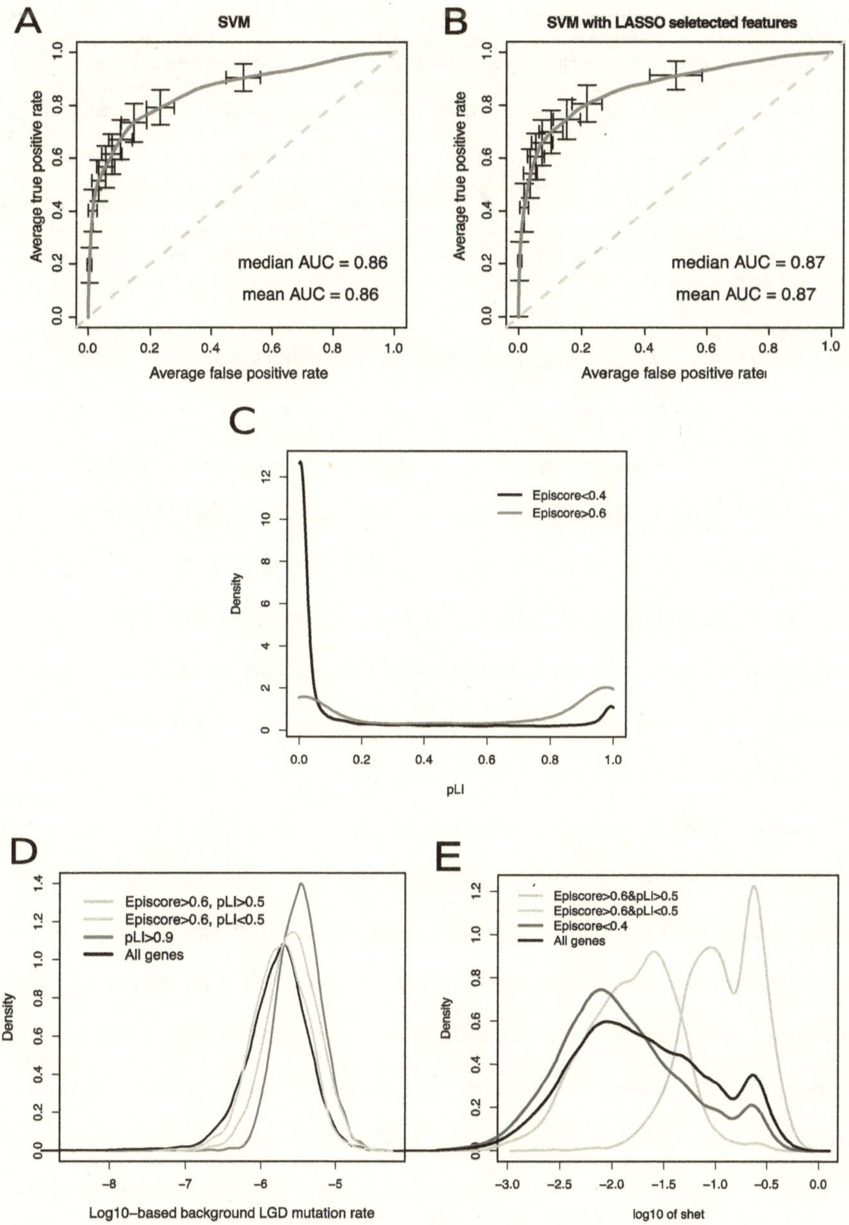

A
SVM
Average true positive rate
Average false positive rate
median AUC = 0.86
mean AUC = 0.86
B
SVM with LASSO seletected features
Average true positive rate
Average false positive rate
median AUC = 0.87
mean AUC = 0.87
C
Density
pLI
Episcore<0.4
Episcore>0.6
D
Density
Episcore>0.6, pLI>0.5
Episcore>0.6, pLI<0.5
pLI>0.9
All genes
Log10-based background LGD mutation rate
E
Density
Episcore>0.6&pLI>0.5
Episcore>0.6&pLI<0.5
Episcore<0.4
All genes
log10 of shet

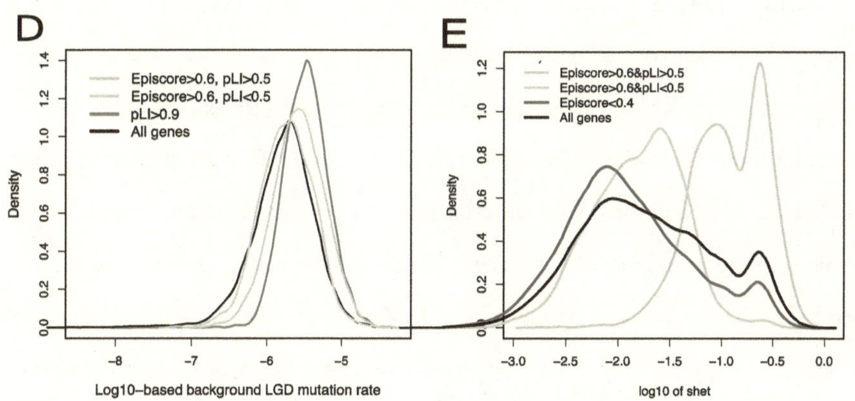

Figure 2.5 Performance of various machine learning approaches and concordance of Episcore with pLI. (A-B) ROC curve of 10-fold cross-validation from applying SVM (A) or SVM with Lasso feature selection (B) to the same epigenetic data as used in the Random Forest model. The red curve is the average of 100 randomized cross-validation runs, with error bar showing standard deviation. (C) pLI distribution of Episcore < 0.4 and Episcore >0.6 genes. The genes with Episcore > 0.6 are much more likely to have pLI values close to 1 than the genes with Episcore < 0.4, and less likely to have pLI values close to 0 than the genes with Episcore <0.4. (D) The distribution of background LGD mutation rate (log10). The genes with Episcore>0.6 and pLI < 0.5 have similar background mutation rate as an average gene, whereas the genes with pLI > 0.5 have higher background mutation rate, and the ones with pLI > 0.9 have even higher background rate. (E) The distribution of Shet: genes with Episcore >0.6 and pLI < 0.5 have intermediate Shet values that are larger than an average gene and smaller than the genes with pLI>0.5. The genes with Episcore < 0.4 on average have reduced Shet compared to other genes.

2.2.3 Episcore better prioritizes of *de novo* LGD variants in developmental disorders

A major goal of predicting haploinsufficiency is to facilitate prioritization of variants identified in genetic studies of developmental disorders. We compared Episcore with pLI scores from ExAC (Lek et al., 2016), S_{het} values (selection coefficient of heterozygous LGD variants) (Cassa et al., 2017), and ranks of mouse heart expression level (Zaidi et al., 2013), using *de novo* LGD variants identified in a recently published whole exome sequencing study DDD (Deciphering Developmental Disorders consortium) of 1,365 trio families with congenital heart disease (CHD) (Sifrim et al., 2016). LGD variants include frameshift, nonsense and canonical splice site mutations. We only included genes with all 4 metrics for comparison, although we note Episcore (19,430 genes) made predictions for more genes than pLI (18,225 genes), S_{het} (17,200 genes) and ranks of mouse heart expression level (17,624 genes, due to loss in orthologue matching). Different predictions are compared by the enrichment rate of variants. For the same number of top-ranked genes by each metric, we calculated the number of LGD variants located in these genes and estimated the number of LGD variants based on background mutation rate (Samocha et al., 2014). Across a wide range of top-ranked genes, Episcore showed larger enrichment than ExAC pLI, S_{het}, or heart expression level (Figure 2.6A and Figure 2.7A). We also applied the same approach to *de novo* synonymous variants identified in the CHD dataset and observed no enrichment (Figure 2.7B). Additionally, we compared these predictions by precision-recall-like curve (PR-like) based on enrichment. Since the total number of positive variants (true disease-causing variants) is unknown, we used estimated number of "true positives" instead of "true positive rate (recall)" in this comparison. For top-ranked genes from each method, the number of true positives were estimated by subtracting expected number of LGD variants based on background mutation rate from the observed in these genes. We measured precision by dividing the estimated number of true positives by the total number of observed LGD variants in these genes. Across a wide range of precision, Episcore consistently showed superior recall compared to pLI, S_{het} and heart expression level (Figure 2.6B) and to earlier methods based on combination of genetic and protein interaction network data (Huang et al., 2010; Steinberg et al., 2015) (Figure 2.7C and D). The performance advantage over other HIS-related score does not change after excluding the genes used in training (Figure 2.7E and F).

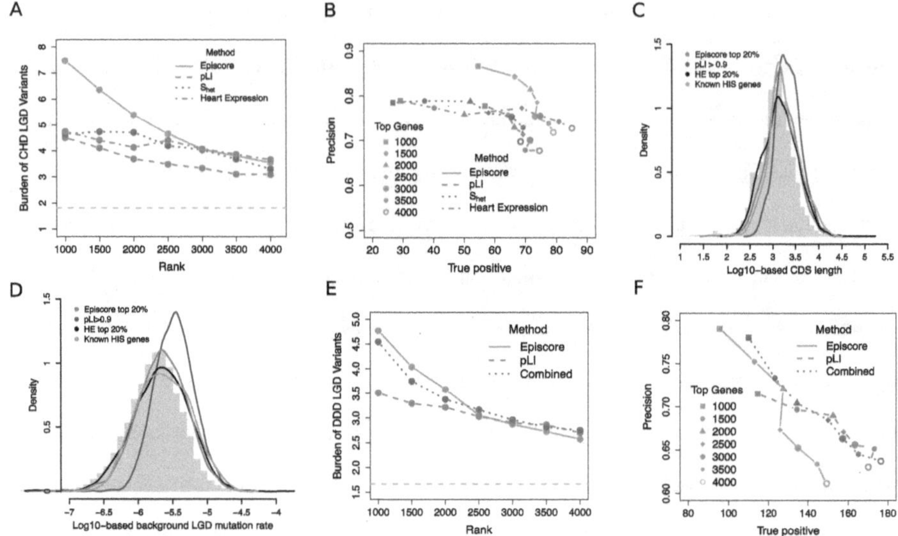

Figure 2.6 Assessment of the performance of Episcore in variant prioritization using *de novo* mutation data. (A-B) Comparison of Episcore, pLI, S_{het} and heart expression level (HE) in variant prioritization using CHD exome sequencing data. In (A), burden refers to the ratio between the number of *de novo* LGD variants observed in top genes ranked by each metric and the number of expected *de novo* LGD variants due to background mutation. Episcore has higher enrichment in top 1000-2500 genes and similar enrichment afterwards. The grey dash line indicates the burden of *de novo* LGD variants in all genes. (B) Precision-recall-like curves. True positive is the difference between the observed and expected *de novo* LGD variants. Precision is calculated by dividing the number of true positives by the number of observed *de novo* LGD variants. The blue curve for Episcore shifts upright than pLI and S_{het}, showing Episcore has better recall with precision and vice versa. (C-D) Episcore has less bias towards genes with longer CDS length (C) or larger background mutation rate (D) than pLI. Grey histogram in the background represents CDS length or mutation rate of all genes in the genome. The blue curve for pLI shifts right, while the curves for Episcore and HE are similar to the distribution of all genes and known HIS genes. (E-F) A combination of Episcore and pLI, the meta-score, has better performance in variant prioritization when benchmarked using DDD exome sequencing data. Meta-score is the output from a logistic regression model, using Episcore and pLI as input. Enrichment, true positive and precision were calculated similarly to (A-B).

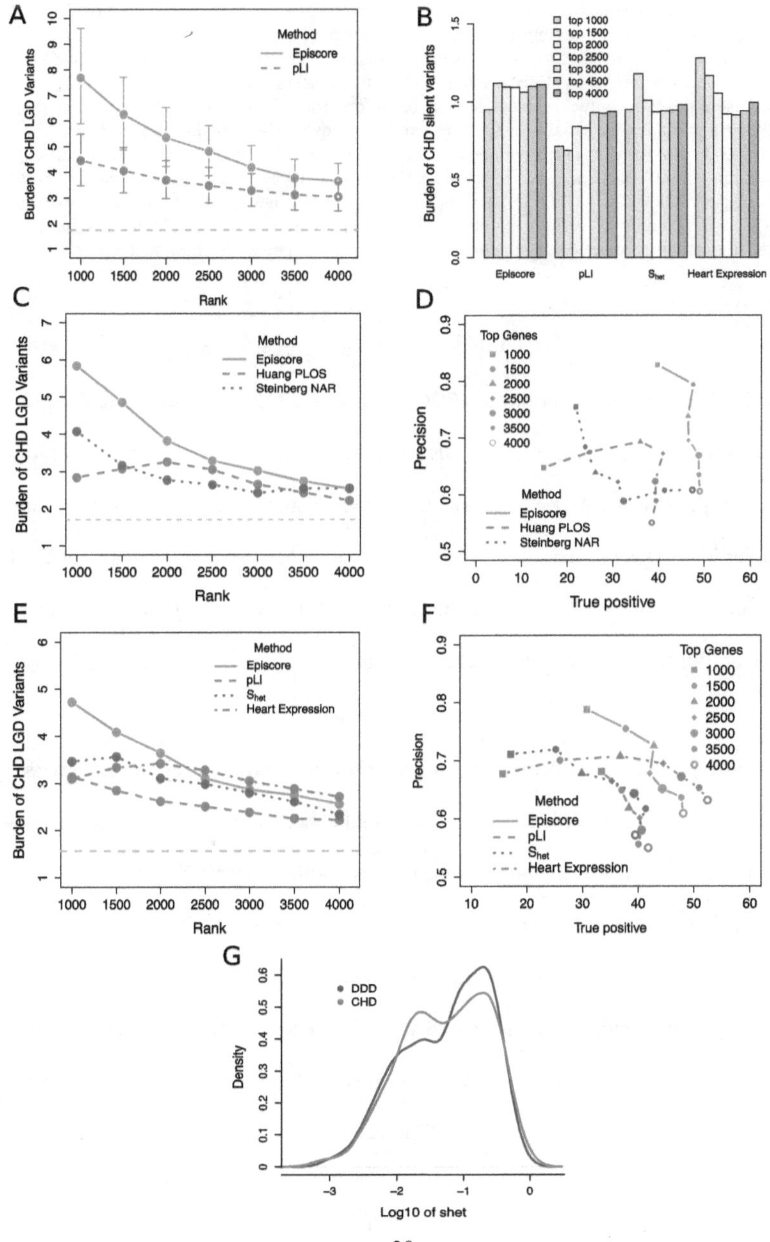

A
Burden of CHD LGD Variants
Method
Episcore
pLI
Rank
B
Burden of CHD silent variants
top 1000
top 1500
top 2000
top 2500
top 3000
top 4500
top 4000
Episcore
pLI
Shet
Heart Expression
C
Burden of CHD LGD Variants
Method
Episcore
Huang PLOS
Steinberg NAR
Rank
D
Precision
Top Genes
1000
1500
2000
2500
3000
3500
4000
Method
Episcore
Huang PLOS
Steinberg NAR
True positive
E
Burden of CHD LGD Variants
Method
Episcore
pLI
Shet
Heart Expression
Rank
F
Precision
Top Genes
1000
1500
2000
2500
3000
3500
4000
Method
Episcore
pLI
Shet
Heart Expression
True positive
G
Density
DDD
CHD
Log10 of shet

Figure 2.7 Using empirical data to benchmark the performance of Episcore in variant prioritization. (A) Comparison of enrichment burden between Episcore and pLI, shown with 95% confidence intervals calculated based on Poisson distribution. (B) Enrichment of CHD silent *de novo* variants is close to 1 regardless of Episcore rank. (C-D) Comparing Episcore to prediction of haploinsufficient genes from two previous studies based on protein interaction networks (Huang et al., 2010; Steinberg et al., 2015), using CHD exome sequencing data. The grey dash line indicates the burden of *de novo* LGD variants acorss the genome. (E-F) Comparison of Episcore, pLI, S_{het} and heart expression level excluding known HIS genes used in training. Episcore achieves better performance than mutation intolerance based metrics. (G) The distribution of S_{het} (log10) of genes that have LGD *de novo* mutations in DDD ID and CHD cases. Overall a larger fraction of genes with mutations in DDD ID cases have high S_{het} values, indicating the disease-causing genes are under more severe selection on average.

We obtained a second CHD WES cohort of 2,645 parent-offspring trios from the Pediatric Cardiac Genomics Consortium (PCGC) (Jin et al., 2017) to emulate a replication design. We used the larger data (PCGC CHD) as discovery and the DDD data as replication. We found that the genes with a single LGD variant in PCGC data and "replicated" with at least one LGD variant in the DDD data have much higher Episcore, than the genes with a singleton LGD in PCGC data or genes with LGD variants in controls (unaffected siblings in Simons Simplex Collection autism study (Krumm et al., 2015))(Figure 2.8).

2.2.4 Episcore provides complementary information to mutation intolerance metrics

Haploinsufficiency predicted by mutation intolerance in a general population (such as ExAC pLI metric) is intrinsically biased towards genes with longer CDS (coding sequence) lengths or higher background mutation rates. Figure 2.6C and D show the distribution of genes with pLI scores > 0.9 shifts towards longer CDS length or higher background mutation rate, as compared to the distribution of known HIS disease risk genes, while top 20% genes ranked by Episcore have similar distribution to known HIS disease risk genes or genes with expression level ranked in top 20% in developing heart (Zaidi et al.).

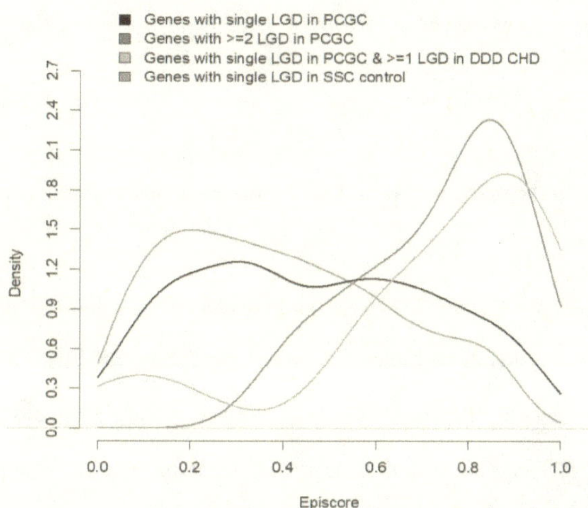

Figure 2.8 Episcore distribution of genes with de novo LGD variants in DDD CHD cohort and PCGC CHD cohort. Data in an earlier version of PCGC CHD cohort is depleted from DDD CHD data due to duplication. The distribution of genes with single LGD variant in PCGC cohort and at least one LGD or D-mis variant in DDD CHD cohort are close to the distribution of genes with multiple LGD variants in PCGC cohort, suggesting that Episcore facilitates discovery of de novo risk genes with only one LGD variant. For comparison, genes with de novo single LGD variant detected from an SSC control cohort have lower Episcore distribution.

Since Episcore and pLI use distinct types of input data, a combination of these two scores might achieve better performance. We obtained de novo mutation data of 4,293 trio families affected by developmental disorders, mostly with intellectual disabilities (DDD ID), from a recent study(McRae et al., 2016). Genes with *de novo* LGD mutations in DDD ID cases are notably under more severe selection than the ones in CHD (Figure 2.7G). We used a logistic regression to integrate Episcore and pLI in this data set. Specifically, we used a total of 45 genes with *de novo* LGD variants in 3 or more probands as positives, and randomly sampled 45 genes from genes with no observed *de novo* LGD variant as negatives to estimate coefficients in the logistic model. Both Episcore and pLI have significant coefficients ($P < 10^{-3}$), supporting these two methods convey complementary information. We found that the resulting meta-score achieved overall better precision and true positives than Episcore or pLI alone (Figure 2.6 E and F), while maintaining similar enrichment burden as good as any method alone in a broad range of gene ranks.

2.2.5 Brain tissues, fetal tissues, and stem cells highly associate with the predicted haploinsufficiency

To evaluate the association of each epigenomic feature to haploinsufficiency, we calculated Spearman correlation coefficients between each feature and Episcore. These correlation coefficients were analyzed in two ways. We first grouped them based on the molecular entities they represent, such that the same epigenomic modification from different tissues would be in one group. Each of the 5 resulting categories has distinct distributions of Spearman correlation coefficients, suggesting different contributions to Episcore (Figure 2.9A). Except for the repressive mark H3K27me3, most of them have larger correlation coefficients than gene expression values, suggesting these features and the model do not merely reflect expression abundance but also epigenomic regulation specific to HIS genes. Measured by mean decrease of Gini index, these groups of features have similar trend in contribution to Episcore prediction (Figure 2.10).

We then grouped correlation coefficients based on tissue and cell types, converted correlation coefficient of each epigenomic modification to a Z-score using the mean and standard deviation across the tissue or cell type, and finally averaged the Z-score of all epigenomic modification for each tissue or cell type. The averaged Z-score represents the importance of this tissue or cell type to haploinsufficiency prediction. In general, stem cells and neural tissues have large average Z-scores (Figure 2.9B). Interestingly, for tissues in the same category, fetal tissues usually have larger average Z-scores than postnatal tissues.

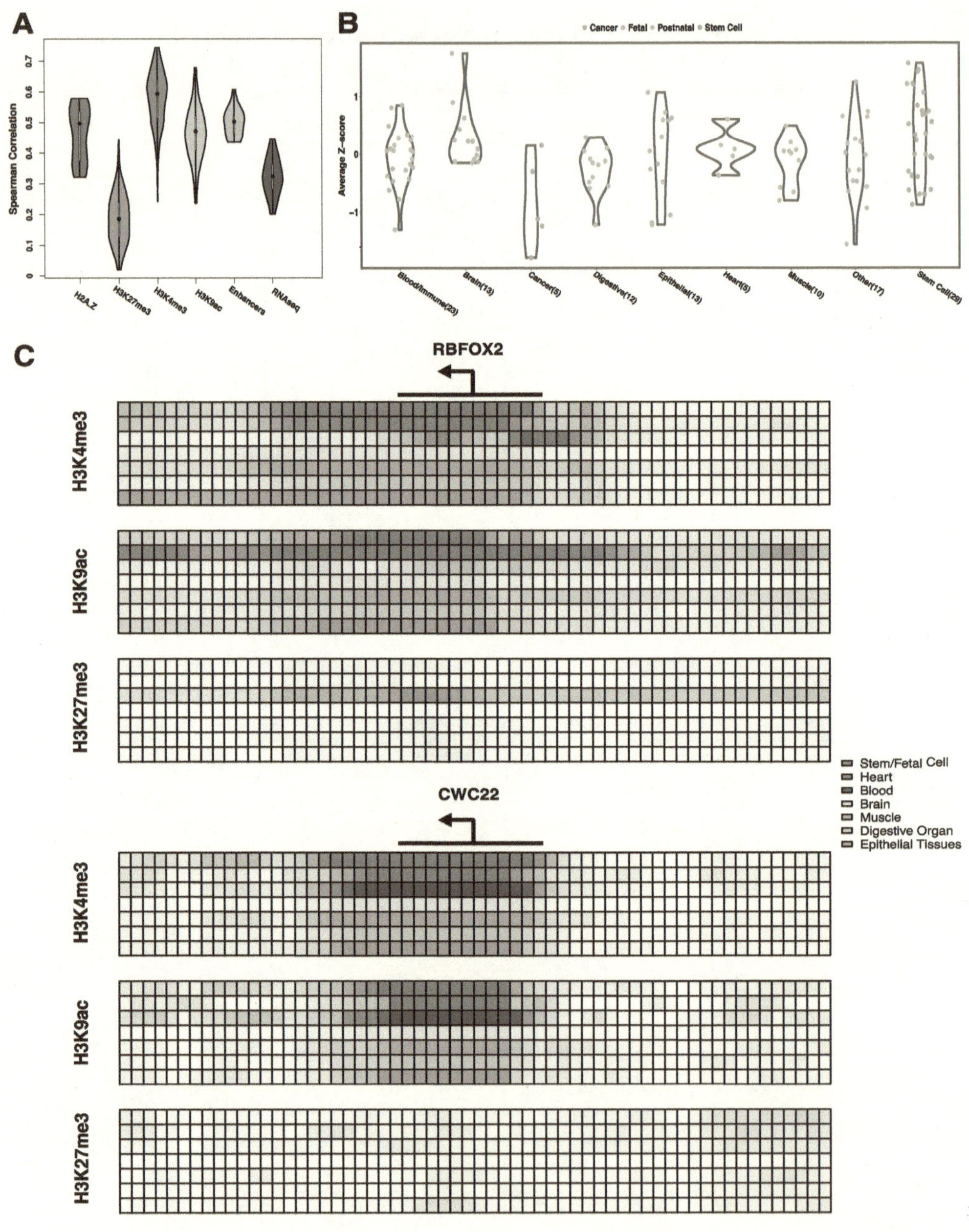
A
Spearman Correlation
0
0.1
0.2
0.3
0.4
0.5
0.6
0.7
H2A.Z
H3K27me3
H3K4me3
H3K9ac
Enhancers
RNAseq
B
Cancer Fetal Postnatal Stem Cell
Average Z-score
1
0
-1
Blood/Immune(23)
Brain(13)
Cancer(5)
Digestive(12)
Epithelial(13)
Heart(5)
Muscle(10)
Other(17)
Stem Cell(29)
C
RBFOX2
H3K4me3
H3K9ac
H3K27me3
CWC22
H3K4me3
H3K9ac
H3K27me3
Stem/Fetal Cell
Heart
Blood
Brain
Muscle
Digestive Organ
Epithelial Tissues

Figure 2.9 Contribution of epigenomic features to Episcore prediction. (A) Spearman correlation between epigenomic feature and Episcore. Features used in the Random Forest model, including H2A.Z, H3K27me3, H3K4me3, H3K9ac and the number of interacting enhancers, all have positive correlation with Episcore. Spearman correlation coefficients between gene expression level, measured in RPKM (reads per kilobase per million reads), and Episcore were also plotted for comparison. (B) The importance of each tissue in generating Episcore is measured by average Z-score, which is converted from Spearman correlation coefficients between epigenomic feature and Episcore. Each dot represents one cell line or tissue type indicated by colors. Stem cells and neural and fetal tissues are the most important tissue and cell types in Episcore prediction. (C) The epigenomic profile of an example HIS gene, *RBFOX2*, and a house-keeping gene, *CWC22*. Each small box represents 100bp region around TSS and the shade of the color reflects averaged fold change of reads between ChIP-seq library and control samples. *RBFOX2* has a broad expansion of epigenomic marks while *CWC22* is not, and *RBFOX2* shows more tissue-specific regulation but *CWC22* has narrow peaks in active marks across all the tissues.

Finally, to illustrate the contribution of different tissues to HIS, we examined in detail the histone modifications around TSS of several known HIS genes. Figure 2.9C show *RBFOX2* and *CWC22*. *RBFOX2* is a CHD risk gene recently discovered through *de novo* LGD variants (Jason Homsy et al.), and it has expansive H3K4me3 and H3K9ac peaks in stem/fetal cells and heart and brain tissues, but not in blood cells. Consistently, it has a reverse pattern in H3K27me3, extensive in blood cells but limited in other tissues. On the contrary, *CWC22,* a known house-keeping gene, shows consistent but narrow peaks of active marks across tissues.

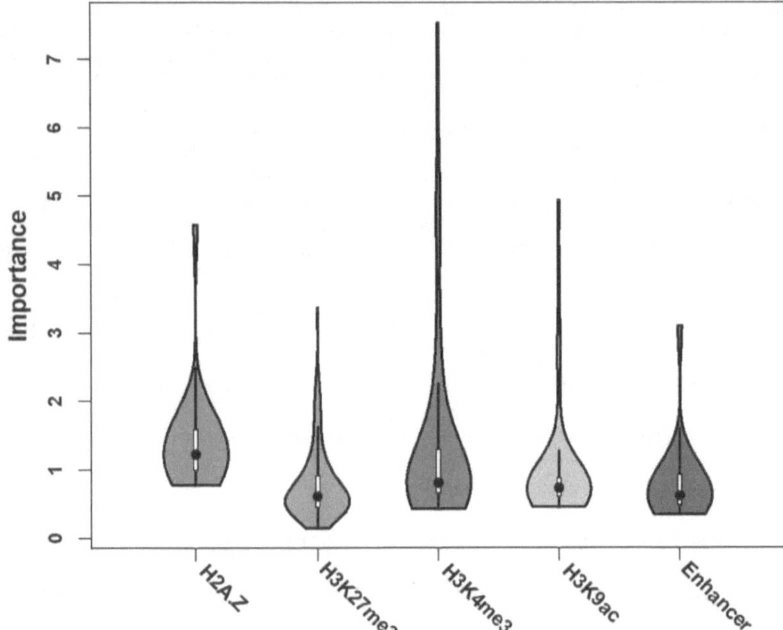

Figure 2.10 The importance (mean decrease of Gini index) of each feature to Episcore prediction. We obtained the importance values from the randomForest R package. Features are grouped by epigenomic molecular entities. For each group, we summarize the distribution of importance metric across cell and tissue types. Active promoter and enhancer features (H3K4me3, H3K9ac, H2A.Z, Enhancer) show higher importance than repressive promoter features (H3K27me3).

2.3 Discussion

In this study we showed there is a strong correlation between epigenomics patterns and gene haploinsufficiency, and developed a computational method (Episcore) to predict HIS using epigenomic features. Episcore had superior yet complementary performance in prioritization of *de novo* LGD variants in congenital heart disease and neurodevelopmental disorders, compared to mutation intolerance metrics such as ExAC pLI (Lek et al.).

Existing HIS prediction methods based on intolerance of mutations have limited statistical power in genes with small transcript size or under less severe negative selection. Network-based methods(Huang et al., 2010) are often biased towards well-studied genes (Steinberg et al., 2015) and pathways. Epigenomic data have several advantages to address these issues: (a) they are orthogonal to genetic mutations, and therefore provide additional information that could improve power; (b) they are much less biased by transcript size, and will be most helpful to predict HIS of genes with short transcripts; (c) the bias with selection coefficient is a reflection of the training data, which empirically is much smaller than mutation intolerance metrics; (d) the ability to generate large amount of data without bias towards well-studied genes. These advantages contribute to the superior performance of Episcore in prioritizing *de novo* LGD variants from exome sequencing studies.

There are likely a variety of mechanisms underlining the correlation of epigenomics patterns and haploinsufficiency. First, broad H3K4me3 peaks contributed most to Episcore prediction of HIS. Broad H3K4me3 peaks are associated with reduced transcriptional noise at cell population and single cell levels (Benayoun et al.), which is likely required to maintain precise expression levels of HIS genes in specific cell types and developmental stages. Second, a previous study found regulatory complexity is required to achieve cell-type specific expression patterns of the lineage-defining genes in hematopoietic differentiation (Gonzalez, Setty, & Leslie). Consistently, we found the number of enhancers interacting with the promotor of a gene is highly correlated with predicted HIS score. Third, many HIS genes are regulators that define cell lineages during differentiation. Bivalent chromatin domains in embryonic stem cells, in which both active marker H3K4me3 and repressor marker H3K27me3 are present, are generally associated with lineage control genes (Vastenhouw & Schier). We observed that H3K27me3 are positively correlated with H3K4me3 in stem cells, and both are correlated with mutation intolerance (Figure 2.1A and C) and Episcore (Figure 2.9A). Finally, we found epigenomic features from stem cells and fetal tissues contribute most to prediction, highlighting the importance of developmental role in determining gene haploinsufficiency.

Our data suggests Episcore is generally better for prioritizing genes with a broader range of selection coefficient or genes with smaller transcript size, whereas pLI performs better for genes under most severe negative selection. Episcore is currently limited by availability and resolution of epigenomic data, especially cell-type specific data from complex tissues or organs such as the brain, and data at various developmental stages. Complex developmental disorders, such as autism, involve a large number of cell types during a broad range of developmental stages. It is critical to generate and integrate more fine-grained epigenomic data from cells of specific types at specific time points in order to improve genetic discoveries in studies of such diseases. We expect such data sets will become available in near future from ongoing projects (Dekker et al.; Psych et al.; Stunnenberg, International Human Epigenome, & Hirst, 2016), and will enable us to improve prediction of HIS and facilitate novel discoveries in genetic studies.

2.4 Material and methods

2.4.1 Collection and Preprocessing of Training Genes

In this study, we used Ensembl release 75 for gene annotation and TSS (transcription start site) locations. All genomic coordinates are based on hg19 human genome assembly. Any non-hg19 coordinates were lifted over to hg19 using UCSC LiftOver tool (https://genome.ucsc.edu/cgi-bin/hgLiftOver). Conversion of gene symbols to Ensembl IDs were based on annotation tables downloaded from Ensembl BioMart.

Positive training set data (curated haploinsufficient genes) were collected from these two sources: (1) haploinsufficent training genes used in previous studies (Dang et al., 2008; Huang et al., 2010) and (2) genes with haploinsufficient score of 3 in ClinGen Dosage Sensitivity Map (http://www.ncbi.nlm.nih.gov/projects/dbvar/clingen/). For the negative training set (curated haplosufficient genes), we used genes deleted in two or more healthy people, based on CNVs detected in 2,026 normal individuals (Shaikh et al., 2009). Only genes with half or more of its length covered by any deletion were considered "deleted" in an individual.

The raw training set may have some false positives and false negatives, as it contained results from automated literature mining that is known to give noisy output. To optimize the performance, we did the following pruning of the raw training set: (1) we only kept protein-coding genes in autosomes, as non-protein-coding genes or genes on sex chromosomes may be under different mechanism of epigenomic regulation; (2) from the positive training set, we removed genes with sufficient contradictory evidence (ExAC pLI ≤ 0.1 and expected loss-of-function variants > 10 (Lek et al.)); and (3) from the negative training set, we removed genes with sufficient contradictory evidence (pLI $\geq$ 0.9 and expected loss-of-function variants > 10). After pruning, the positive training set has 287 genes and the negative training set has 717 genes. The full list of training genes is available in Supplementary Table 2.1.

2.4.2 Preprocessing of Epigenomic Feature Data

The uniformly processed peak calling results of Roadmap and ENCODE projects were downloaded from http://egg2.wustl.edu/roadmap/web_portal/processed_data.html. For promoter features (H2A.Z, H3K27me3, H3K4me3, and H3K9ac), "GappedPeaks" were used to allow for broad domains of ChIP-seq signal. The assignment of a GapppedPeak to a gene follows these steps in order: (1) for each gene, only TSS of Ensembl canonical transcripts were used. (2) assigned a GappedPeak to a TSS if the GappedPeak overlaps with the upstream 5kb to downstream 1kb region around the TSS. This definition of basal cis-regulatory region around promoter follows GREAT tool (McLean et al., 2010). Assigning one GappedPeak to multiple TSS was allowed. (3) For TSS having more than 1 GappedPeak assigned, kept the closest one. (4) For genes with multiple TSS and hence multiple assigned GappedPeaks, kept the longest GappedPeak. After these four steps, if one gene had been associated with a GappedPeak, then we used the width of the peak as an epigenomic feature in the following machine learning models. If a gene had no associated GappedPeak, then the peak width is 0.

To calculate the number of interacting enhancers of a gene, we used two approaches. In a naïve approach, we counted peaks of ChIP-seq signals that are associated with enhancers. The ChIP-seq signals we used include H3K4me1, H3K27ac and DNase I hypersensitivity site, and each ChIP signal was counted and recorded separately. We used "NarrowPeak" instead of "GappedPeak" in the counting to better estimate the number of interacting enhancers, as enhancer regions are not long and GappedPeak has the risk of merging nearby ChIP-seq signals. For each gene, we counted peaks in (a) the surrounding TAD (Topologically Associated Domain), based on TADs reported in (Dixon et al., 2012); or (b) +/- 20kb of each TSS (Only TSSs of Ensembl canonical transcripts were used. For genes with multiple TSS and thus several numbers of interacting enhancers, we kept the largest one). In a more advanced approach, we adapted EpiTensor (Zhu et al., 2016) to infer gene-enhancer relationship. We made a few changes when using EpiTensor: (a) we used normalized coverage of ChIP-seq signal instead of raw coverage in Zhu et al. 2016 (Zhu et al.); (b) we used the coverage of H3K27ac, H3K27me3, H3K36me3, H3K4me1, H3K4me3, H3K9me3, DNase I and RNA-seq as input for EpiTensor to balance between more input data types and more cell types included, as not every cell type has all these histone modifications characterized. The number of data types included are fewer than the ones used in Zhu et al. 2016 (Zhu et al.), but it could still achieve desirable performance (personal communications); (c) we used enhancer annotation from 15-state chromHMM (http://egg2.wustl.edu/roadmap/web_portal/chr_state_learning.html#core_15state), while the original EpiTensor paper (Zhu et al.) used results of an earlier version. Based on the output of EpiTensor, which predicts enhancer-promoter pairs, we counted the number of interacting enhancers for each gene in various tissues.

Finally, the results of peak width and number of interacting enhancers were consolidated into a matrix, with each row being a gene and each column representing a combination of a tissue and a data type, e.g. "H3K4me3 peak width in fetal heart". One combination of a tissue and a data type was referred to as one epigenomic feature. This matrix was used as input for machine learning models described in the following section.

2.4.3 Machine learning approaches to predict haploinsufficiency

We applied several machine learning approaches, including Random Forest, Support Vector Machine (SVM) and SVM with LASSO feature selection. Random Forest was implemented using R package "randomForest". SVM was implemented using R package "e1071". LASSO was implemented using R package "glmnet", with alpha value equal to 1. For each machine learning method, we assessed the performance based on 100 runs of 10-fold cross-validation. In each run, 10% of the training genes were randomly selected and left out to form a test set for validation. The remaining data were used to train the model, after which the test set was used to calculate model sensitivity and specificity. We used R package "ROCR" to make a ROC curve based on the 100 runs and calculated AUC values.

Finally, we used all training genes used to train the model, and then estimate the probabilities of being positive (i.e. probabilities of being HIS) for all genes. The whole process was repeated 30 times and we took the arithmetic mean of the 30 sets of probabilities as the final results.

2.4.4 Comparing Episcore and other metrics in variant prioritization

We used two approaches to compare Episcore and other metrics in variant prioritization, based on "enrichment of *de novo* LGD variants", estimated "number of true-positives" and "precision". The formula to calculate these three statistics are as follows.

For any gene $\boldsymbol{i}$, the number of expected *de novo* LGD variants in each gene, $\boldsymbol{E_i}$, was calculated as:

$$\boldsymbol{E_i = 2 \times N \times r_i}$$

where $\boldsymbol{N}$ is the number of cases in the sequencing cohort and $\boldsymbol{r_i}$ is gene-specific LGD mutation rate. LGD variants include nonsense, frameshift and canonical splice site mutations. The background mutation rate per gene of each mutation type was obtained from Samocha et al. 2014 (Samocha et al.). For each gene, $\boldsymbol{r_i}$ is the sum of background mutation rate of nonsense, frameshift and canonical splice site mutations.

For a set of genes, the enrichment of *de novo* LGD variants, $\boldsymbol{D}$, was calculated as:

$$\boldsymbol{D = \frac{M}{\sum_i E_i}}$$

where $\boldsymbol{M}$ is the total number of observed *de novo* LGD variants in this gene set. In this study, we used results from two whole exome sequencing studies on congenital heart disease (Jason

Homsy et al., 2015; Sifrim et al., 2016) and another whole exome sequencing study on various developmental disorders (McRae et al., 2016).

For any gene set, the number of true positives, ***TP***, was calculated as:

$$\boldsymbol{TP = M - \sum_i E_i}$$

For any gene set, the precision (positive predictive value), ***PPV***, was calculated as:

$$\boldsymbol{PPV = \frac{M - \sum_i E_i}{M}}$$

For each metric (Episcore, pLI, etc.), a series of top-ranked genes were selected, such as top 500 genes, top 2000 genes, etc. In the first approach, enrichment of *de novo* LGD variants, ***D***, was calculated for any set of top-ranked genes, and then enrichment values were plotted and compared, as shown in Figure 2.6A. In the second approach, the number of true positives, ***TP***, and the precision (true discovery rate), ***PPV***, were calculated for any set of top-ranked genes. ***TP*** and ***PPV*** were plotted and compared, as shown in Figure 2.6B. If the number of all true positives (*N*) in a study is known, we can calculate recall as *R* = *TP*/*N*. Although *N* is generally unknown, it is a constant; therefore, *TP* is proportional to *R*. In this study, we use TP as a proxy of recall.

To examine the utility of Episcore in prioritizing genes with only one LGD mutation, we utilized two independent Congenital Heart Disease (CHD) cohorts: DDD (Deciphering Developmental Disorders consortium) CHD (Sifrim et al., 2016) and PCGC (Pediatric Cardiac Genomics Consortium) CHD (Jin et al., 2017). Both these studies included trios from an earlier CHD study (Zaidi et al., 2013) to increase detection power. To avoid duplication, we removed these earlier trios from DDD CHD data.

2.4.5 Epigenomic features critical in the prediction

We calculated a Spearman correlation coefficient between each epigenomic feature and Episcore. One epigenomic feature here corresponds to a data type (like H3K4me3 peak width) in certain tissue/cell type (e.g. fetal heart). To examine which data types are more important, we plotted these Spearman correlation coefficients by data type, e.g. correlation coefficients from H3K4me3 peak width were plotted in one section. To examine what tissue/cell types are more important, we calculated averaged z-score for each tissue/cell type. The average z-score is calculated following these two steps: (1) we converted every Spearman correlation coefficient to a Z-score using mean and standard deviation specific to each data type and (2) for each tissue/cell type, we averaged the Z-scores from various data types.

Chapter 3: Dissecting Autism Genetic Risk Using Single-cell RNA-seq Data

3.1 Introduction

Autism spectrum disorder (autism) is a phenotypically heterogeneous developmental disorder, affecting 1 in 59 children in the United States (Baio et al., 2018). Earlier studies have shown a strong genetic basis for autism with up to 90% concordance between monozygotic twins (Bailey et al., 1995; Rosenberg et al., 2009) and 10-fold higher chance for younger sibling to be diagnosed with autism if there is an older affected sibling (Constantino, Zhang, Frazier, Abbacchi, & Law, 2010; Ronemus, Iossifov, Levy, & Wigler, 2014). Simulations estimate one thousand autism risk genes with large effect (Iossifov et al., 2014); however, currently only about 100 known risk genes (Abrahams et al., 2013) have robust evidence from recent studies (De Rubeis et al., 2014; Iossifov et al., 2014; Turner et al., 2016). These known risk genes only account for less than 5% of autism cases (Krumm, O'Roak, Shendure, & Eichler, 2014). Therefore, it is critically important to identify new risk genes. However, the identification of new risk genes based on statistical evidence is limited by lack of power due to sample sizes.

A general approach to improve the power for detecting risk genes is to use prior knowledge and functional genomic data to predict plausibility of candidate risk genes. Previous studies have implemented network-based methods utilizing genotype-phenotype associations (Baio et al., 2018; Chang, Gilman, Chiang, Sanders, & Vitkup, 2015; Gilman et al., 2011), protein-protein physical interactions (O'Roak et al., 2012), brain-specific functional interactions (Krishnan et al., 2016) and gene coexpression networks (Parikshak et al., 2013; Willsey et al., 2013). We previously developed a semi-supervised method using cell-type specific expression profiles from mouse bulk microarray data based on Principle Component Analysis (PCA) (C. Zhang & Shen, 2017). One advantage of using cell-type specific expression is the ability to jointly infer plausible risk genes and cell types that are correlated with risk plausibility, potentially improving the understanding of the disease mechanism. Our method was limited by the lack of spatiotemporal cell-type information from developing brains and the species difference between mouse and human. Recent studies have developed machine learning approaches to classify autism risk genes with human brain expression data (Brueggeman, Koomar, & Michaelson, 2018; Lin, Rajadhyaksha, Potash, & Han, 2018), but are still limited by the resolution of data in cell types or developmental stages pertinent to the disease.

With the motivation to identify new risk genes for autism, here we developed a supervised machine learning method based on gradient boosting trees, "A-risk" (Autism risk), that can learn known risk genes' expression patterns in single-cell transcriptomics of human fetal midbrain and prefrontal cortex, to then predict the plausibility of any gene being an autism risk gene. We hypothesize that autism risk genes have distinct spatiotemporal expression signatures in developing human brain in neurotypicals. When comparing A-risk to other metrices or methods in prioritizing risk variants, we observed better performance of A-risk in prioritizing candidate risk variants using *de novo* variant data of 8838 trios from recent publications(R. Chen et al., 2017; Feliciano et al., 2019; Iossifov et al., 2014; Satterstrom et al., 2020; Takata et al., 2018; Yuen et al., 2017). Furthermore, we showed that A-risk and gene mutation intolerance metrics(Lek et al., 2016) can be combined to improve prior estimation in an empirical Bayesian model and enables identification of additional novel risk genes. Finally, we investigated the cell type specific expression patterns in adult brain of known and novel autism risk genes and found that they are highly expressed in deep-layer excitatory neurons in adult human cortex, suggesting the association of deep excitatory neurons in cortex to the etiology of autism.

3.2 Results

3.2.1 Single-cell expression pattern is correlated with autism risk

We obtained two single-cell RNA-seq data sets from human fetal midbrain and prefrontal cortex. The midbrain data are mostly from the first trimester (La Manno et al., 2016), while the prefrontal cortex data are mostly from the second trimester (Zhong et al., 2018). Previous studies have suggested the role of prefrontal cortex (Amaral, Schumann, & Nordahl, 2008; Geschwind, 2011; Rubenstein, 2011; Voineagu et al., 2011) and midbrain dopamine system (D'Ardenne et al., 2012; Ott & Nieder, 2019; Ranganath & Jacob, 2016). On average, 2302 and 4503 genes per cell are detected in the midbrain and the prefrontal cortex data, respectively

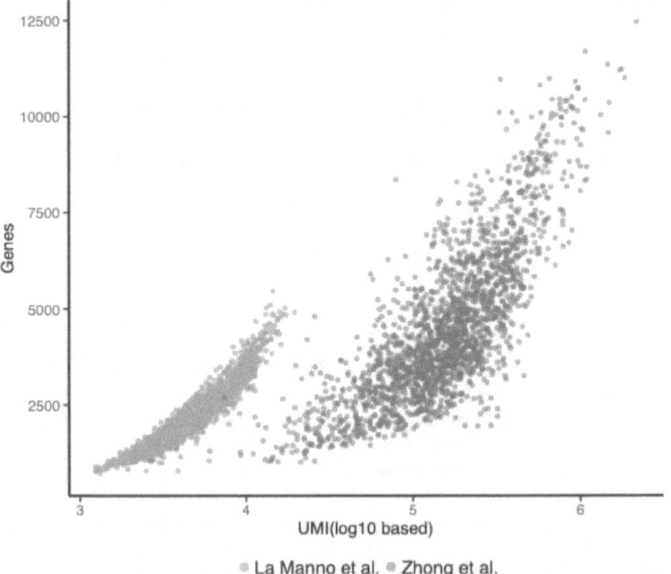

Figure 3.1 Quality of single cell RNA-seq data. The number of log10 based UMIs in each cell from the two data sets against the number of genes detected. The detected genes are defined as genes with larger or equal to 1 UMI. The midbrain data has more genes detected than the prefrontal cortex data given the same number of UMIs.

(Figure 3.1). We obtained the cell type labels from original publications, and then define the expression level of a gene in a cell type as the fraction of cells with ≥1 UMIs (Unique Molecular Identifiers) in the cell type at a certain developmental time point. The feature set of our data is the combination of cell types and developmental time points (Supplementary Table 3.1).

To investigate temporal and cell type specific expression pattern of autism risk genes, we collected 88 known autism risk genes from the SFARI (Simons Foundation Autism Research Initiative) Gene database (Abrahams et al., 2013) (released version on 08/29/2019, score 1 or 2), which are genes strongly implicated in autism based on expert curation from the literature. We also obtained 154 genes with at least 1 *de novo* LGD (likely-gene disrupting) variant in unaffected siblings from an exome-sequencing study(Iossifov et al., 2014) (Supplementary Table 3.2), representing non-risk genes with random *de novo* mutations. Known risk genes tend to have a wide range of average expression level in both data sets, while non-risk genes have lower average expression (Figure 3.2A). We performed PCA (Principle Component Analysis) of these two groups of genes using expression level from the single cell data sets. The first component partially separates known risk genes and non-risk genes (Figure 3.2B). This is consistent with previous findings using bulk RNA microarray data from mouse brain (C. Zhang & Shen, 2017).

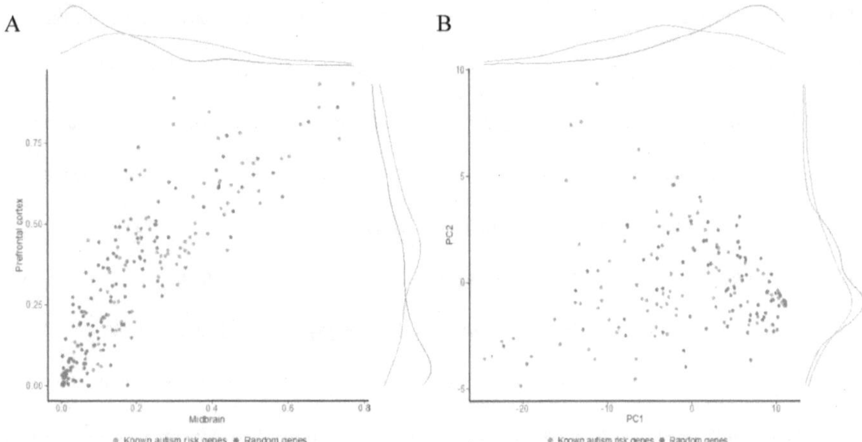

Figure 3.2. Different expression pattern of known autism risk genes and random genes in fetal midbrain and prefrontal cortex. (A) The expression distribution of known autism risk genes and random genes in fetal midbrain and prefrontal cortex. (B) PCA analysis of fraction expression of known autism risk genes and random genes. The density plots along axes shows the difference of known risk genes and random genes in expression level or PCA scores.

To leverage the temporal and cell type specific expression pattern of known autism risk genes, we developed a supervised machine learning method, "A-risk", to predict plausibility of being an autism risk gene for all protein-coding genes (Supplementary Table 3.3). A-risk is based on gradient boosting. We train the model using 88 known autism risk genes as positives and the 154 non-risk genes as negatives. Figure 3.3A shows the overall workflow of A-risk.

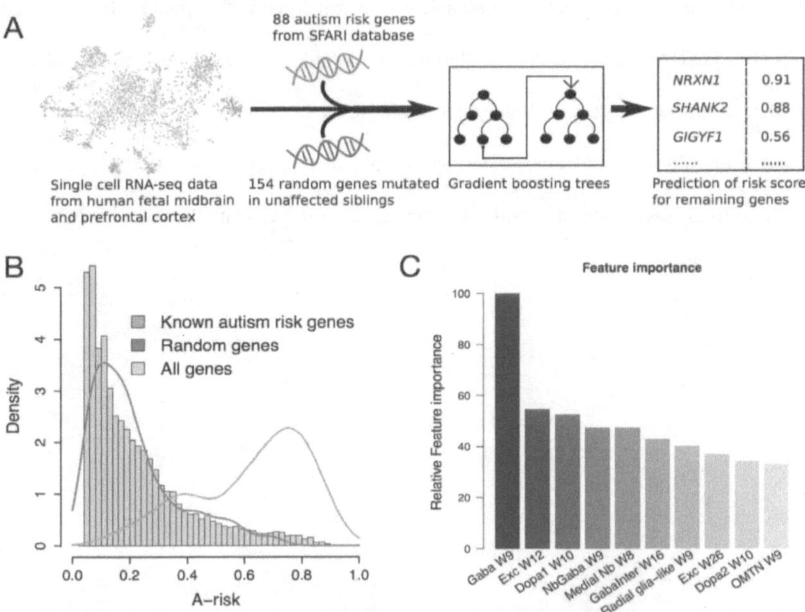

Figure 3.3 A-risk, a gradient boosting tree model to estimate plausibility of being risk genes of autism from single-cell RNA-seq data. (A) A flowchart of the method. (B) A-risk score distribution. A-risk of all genes in the genome are shown in the histogram in gray. The distribution of A-risk of known autism risk genes and randomly mutated genes, which are positive and negative training sets in A-risk model respectively, are shown as orange and purple density curves. A-risk score 0.4 is where the positives and negatives show separation. (C) "Feature importance" derived from the gradient boosting trees model showing cell types from both midbrain late first trimester and prefrontal cortex second trimester make substantial contribution to the prediction. The y-axis is the relative important of each feature against the max, which is GABAergic neurons in midbrain at week 9. W, week. Gaba, GABAergic neurons. Exc, excitatory neurons. Dopa, Dopaminergic neurons. NbGaba, neuroblast GABAergic. Nb, neuroblast. Gabalnter, GABAergic interneurons. OMTN, oculomotor and trochlear nucleus.

Five-fold cross-validation during training achieves an average AUC (Area Under Curve) of ROC (Receiver Operating Characteristic) curves at 0.77 (Figure 3.4). A-risk score distribution shows a large separation of known risk genes and non-risk genes (Figure 3.3B). We chose A-risk 0.4, corresponding to top 2642 ranked genes, as a recommended cutoff for analysis where a binary stratification of genes is needed.

We quantify the contribution of cell types to A-risk prediction by feature importance, a score for each feature measuring how valuable it is in constructing the model. The top ranked cell types are GABAergic neurons in midbrain at week 9, dopaminergic neurons in midbrain at week 10 and prefrontal cortex excitatory neurons at week 12 (Figure 3.3C). Overall, cell types from both midbrain late first trimester and prefrontal cortex second trimester made substantial contribution to the prediction. The full list of feature importance from the model is available in Supplementary Table 3.4.

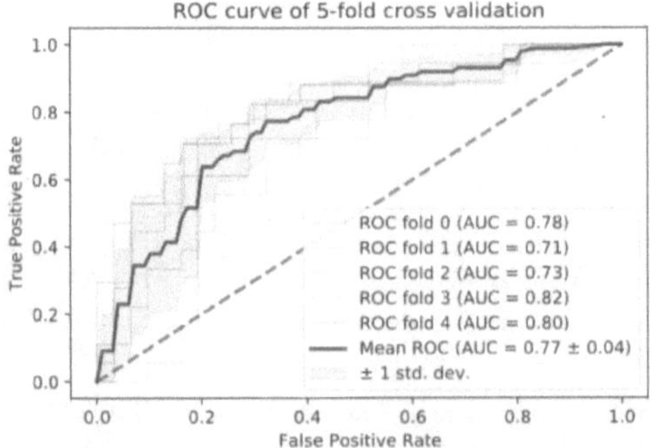

Figure 3.4 Training of A-risk: performance in cross-validation and importance of cell types and time points to the model. ROC curves of 5-fold cross validation using training data, where the training samples are divided as 80% for training and 20% for validation. The blue curve is the average of the 5 curves and the grey band in the background marks the interval between the left and right first standard deviation.

3.2.2 A-risk improves prioritization of *de novo* variants in autism cases

To investigate if A-risk can prioritize *de novo* risk variants detected from exome or genome sequencing studies, we compiled *de novo* likely gene-disrupting (LGD) variants of 8838 trios from recent published studies (R. Chen et al., 2017; Feliciano et al., 2019; Iossifov et al., 2014; Satterstrom et al., 2020; Takata et al., 2018; Yuen et al., 2017) (Table 3.1). We calculated enrichment rate of LGD *de novo* variants in a gene set by the observed number of variants divided by the expected number estimated from background mutation rate models (Carlson et al., 2018; Samocha et al., 2014) (Table 3.2). The enrichment rate for all genes excluding known risk genes is 1.4, suggesting there are additional risk genes that harbor *de novo* LGD variants. When further selecting genes by A-risk ≥0.4, the enrichment rate reaches 2.1 (p-value=1.3e-32, Poisson test), showing that A-risk can increase the signal-to-noise ratio in prioritized candidate risk genes.

Table 3.1 Summary of publication sources of *de novo* variants data.

Cohort label	Number of unique cases	Publication
ASC	3625	(Satterstrom et al., 2020)
De Rubies	421	(De Rubeis et al., 2014)
SSC	2501	(Iossifov et al., 2014)
SPARK pilot	465	(Feliciano et al., 2019)
MSSNG	1529	(Yuen et al., 2017)
JPASD	232	(Takata et al., 2018)
ACE	65	(R. Chen et al., 2017)
Total	8838	

Table 3.2 A-risk improves prioritization of *de novo* LGD variant in autism cases (n=8836).

	Observed number of variants	Expected	Enrichment Rate	P-value
All genes (N=18663)	1341	784	1.7	3e-73
Excluding known risk genes (N=18575)	1114	774	1.4	9e-31
A-risk≥0.4, excluding known risk genes (N=2566)	313	148	2.1	1e-32

To further assess the utility of A-risk in prioritizing novel risk genes, we compute enrichment and precision-recall like curves and compare with other methods. The precision-recall like curves compare the utility of each method in prioritizing true risk variants(Carlson et al., 2018; Samocha et al., 2014). With each method, we rank all genes. In all genes above a certain rank threshold, we estimate the number of detected true risk variants ("positives") by the difference of observed number of variants ("detected positives") and expected number. The total number of true positives is unknown, but it is a constant independent of methods. Therefore, the estimated number of true positives is a proxy of recall. The estimated precision is the number of detected true positives divided by the total number of detected positives. Besides the *de novo* LGD variants we used for Table 3.1, we included deleterious missense (D-mis) variants defined by REVEL score (Ioannidis et al., 2016) ≥0.5 in the following analysis. In addition, all known risk genes used in model training are excluded from analysis. We compared A-risk with mouse brain bulk expression ranks at E9.5 (J. Homsy et al., 2015), ExAC pLI (Lek et al., 2016), and the baseline where the corresponding estimates are calculated in all protein-coding genes (excluding known risk genes). A-risk achieves consistently higher enrichment from the top 2000 to top 4000 ranked genes compared to others and significantly higher than the genome baseline (Figure 3.5A). At the 2500 top rank, roughly corresponding to A-risk score 0.4, A-risk achieves better precision than other metrices and prioritizes almost half of total *de novo* variants with a relatively high precision (0.46), a 64% improvement from the genome-wide baseline (precision=0.28) (Figure 3.5B). Furthermore, in non-constrained genes (pLI<0.9), A-risk shows significantly higher enrichment and better precision compared to mouse brain expression levels (Figure 3.5C and D), indicating A-risk is complementary to pLI with the potential to optimize risk gene discovery, especially among non-constraint genes. We also compared A-risk with other recent methods aimed to find novel autism risk genes, such as D-score (C. Zhang & Shen, 2017) and Krishnan 2016 (Krishnan et al., 2016) (Figure 3.6). A-risk again shows superior performance in enrichment, precision and true positives from top 1500 to top 4000 ranks of the three methods (Figure 3.6A and B), and particularly in non-constrained genes (Figure 3.6C and D).

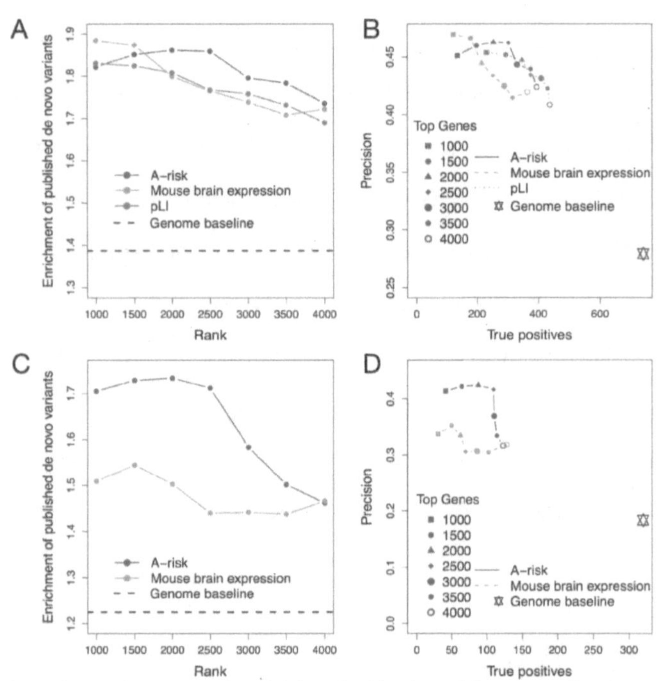

Figure 3.5 Superior performance of A-risk in prioritization of *de novo* variants at top 2500 ranks, especially in non-constraint genes. A-B, comparison of A-risk to mouse brain expression level, pLI and genome baseline in prioritization of *de novo* LGD and D-mis variants among top genes ranked by each individual metrics, excluding known risk genes used in A-risk training. D-mis is defined by REVEL score ≥ 0.5. The *de novo* variant data is compiled from 8838 published trios of exome sequencing studies. (A) Enrichment is the ratio of observed number of *de novo* variants to the expected number of *de novo* variants estimated by background mutation rate in top ranks, ranging from top 1000 to top 4000 genes. (B) Precision and true positives compared in top ranks. True positives, which are the difference value between observed number of de novo variants and the expected number, represent the recall since the true number of total causal variants is unknown. Precision is computed as dividing true positives by the observed number. Genome baseline is the grey star in the plot. C-D, comparison of A-risk to mouse brain expression level and genome baseline in prioritizing de novo variants in non-constraint genes with pLI<0.9, excluding known risk genes. pLI is excluded from the comparison because it is used in stratifying non-constraint genes. (C) Enrichment compared in top ranks by each metric. (D) Precision and true positives comparison.

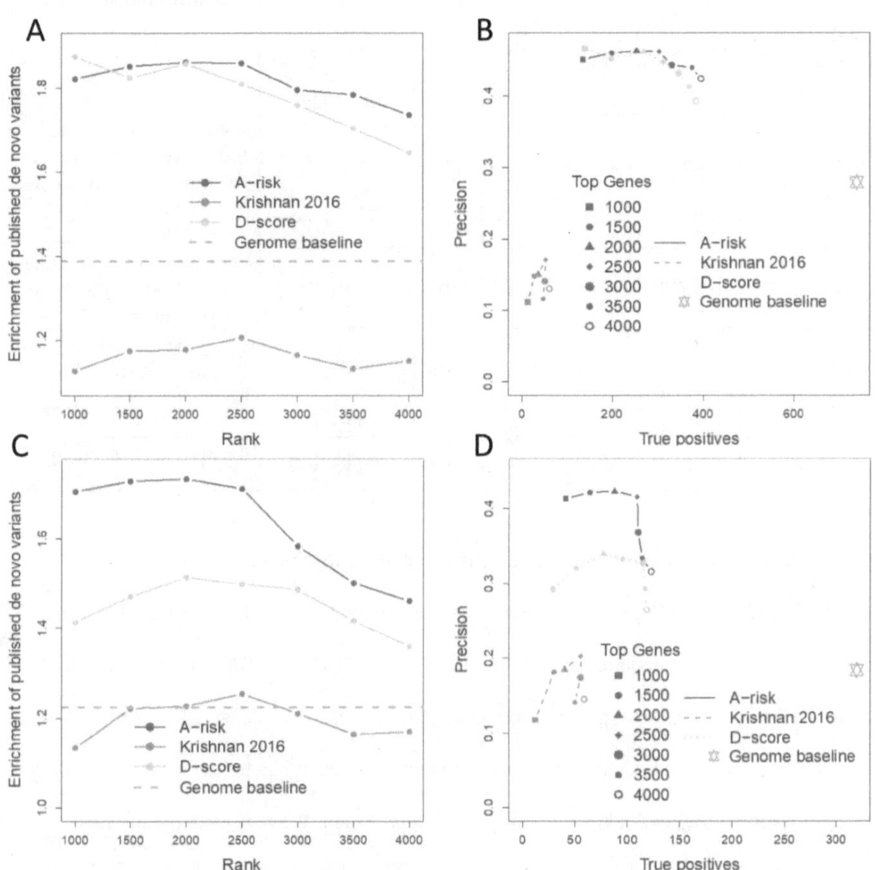

Figure 3.6 A-risk has better performance than other two methods in prioritizing de novo variants. A-B, Compare A-risk to Krishnan 2016(Krishnan et al., 2016) and D-score(C. Zhang & Shen, 2017) in enrichment, precision and true positives of de novo LGD and D-mis variants prioritized in top ranks by each method, excluding all known risk genes. C-D, Compare the three methods in non-constraint genes stratified by pLI < 0.9, excluding all known genes.

Table 3.3 Notable candidate risk genes by stratified extTADA analysis.

Gene Symbol	pLI	A-risk	Gene quadrant	# of LoF, Dmis	FDR	NDD significant genes (Kaplanis et al., 2020)	Additional support
NR2F1	1	0.68	A	1, 1	0.07	TRUE	Bosch-Boonstra-Schaaf Optic Atrophy Syndrome with autistic manifestation (C. A. Chen et al.)
NR4A2	1	0.43	A	1, 1	0.09	TRUE	Levy 2018 (Levy et al.)
CLCN4	1	0.59	A	0, 3	0.015	TRUE	Raynaud-Claes syndrome (OMIM 300114) with autistic features
PRKAR1B	0.18	0.43	C	1, 2	0.06	TRUE	Additional damaging variants in Ruzzo 2019 (Ruzzo et al.)
GIGYF1	0	0.56	C	5, 0	1e-5	TRUE	
HNRNPU	1	0.48	A	1, 1	0.09	TRUE	Mosaic mutations (Lim et al.)

3.2.3 A-risk informs prior estimation in autism risk gene discovery

TADA and extTADA (X. He et al., 2013; Nguyen et al., 2017) are empirical Bayesian methods used in previous genetic studies of autism(De Rubeis et al., 2014; Satterstrom et al., 2020) to identify candidate risk genes based on burden of *de novo* variants. A key feature of such empirical Bayesian method is that it estimates parameters of priors, including mean relative risk ($\boldsymbol{R}$) and prior probability ($\boldsymbol{\pi}$) of being a risk gene, from the data. We reasoned that metrics associated with plausibility of autism risk, such as A-risk and gene constraint (pLI), could be used to improve prior estimation in an empirical Bayesian framework. To this end, we stratified a total of 18663 protein-coding genes by A-risk score 0.4 and pLI cutoff 0.9, resulting in 4 quadrants of genes (Figure 3.7A): 1195 constrained genes with high A-risk score (quadrant A), 1842 constrained genes with low A-risk score (quadrant B), 1444 non-constrained genes with high A-risk score (quadrant C) and 14182 non-constrained genes with low A-risk score (quadrant

D); then we estimated prior parameters by extTADA in each quadrant of genes, using previously reported *de novo* LGD and D-mis variant data from 8838 trios(R. Chen et al., 2017; Feliciano et al., 2019; Iossifov et al., 2014; Satterstrom et al., 2020; Takata et al., 2018; Yuen et al., 2017). Consistent with previous simulation(Iossifov et al., 2014), in unstratified analysis, π is about 0.04, corresponding to 750 risk genes in total. In stratified analysis, π decreases from quadrant A to quadrant D (Figure 3.7B). Constrained genes stratified by A-risk ≥0.4 in quadrant A have

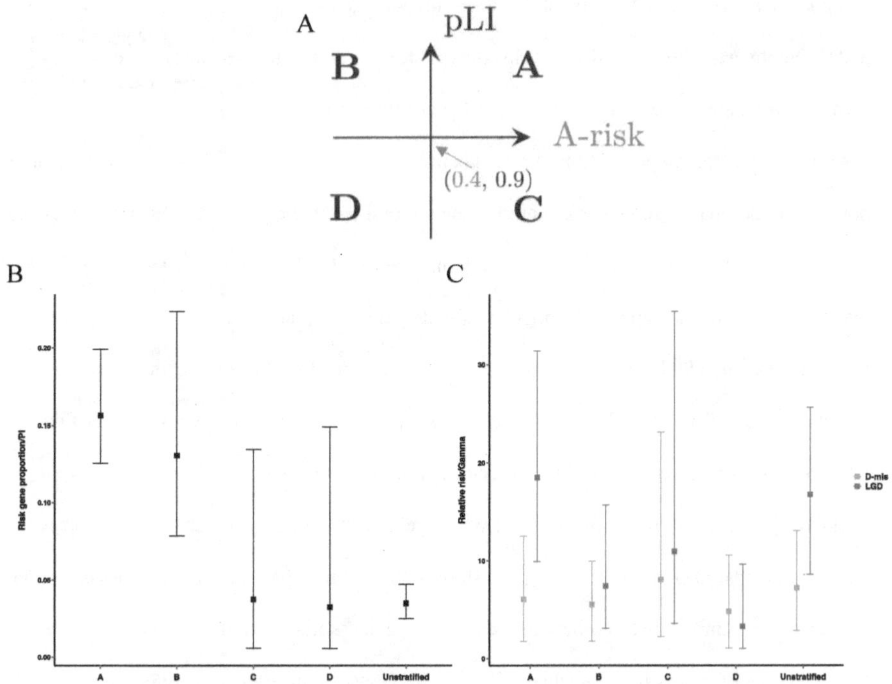

Figure 3.7. Prior estimation in stratified extTADA analysis. (A). gene groups defined by pLI and A-risk: A: pLI≥0.9 and A-risk≥ 0.4; B: pLI≥0.9 and A-risk <0.4; C: pLI<0.9 and A-risk≥0.4; D: pLI<0.9 and A-risk<0.4. (B). Risk gene proportions (π) in stratified gene groups estimated from MCMC. Modes are indicated by small boxes in the middle and the upper and lower bars indicate 95% confidence intervals. (C). Relative risks (γ) of genes in each stratified group estimated from MCMC. Relative risks estimated separately from LGD and D-mis variant data, labeled by purple and orange respectively.

greater π and R than genes with low A-risk scores in quadrant B (Figure 3.7C). Genes in quadrant C and D have similar π, but quadrant C genes have a substantially greater R that D genes. Overall, A-risk informs the estimation of those priors in both constrained and non-constrained genes.

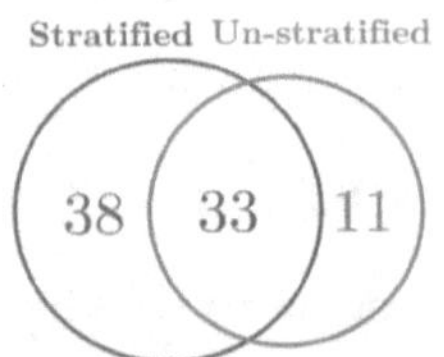

Figure 3.8 Stratified extTADA analysis by A-risk and pLI identifies more candidate risk genes of autism. The numbers in the Venn diagram show the number of genes identified by stratified analysis exclusively (38), by un-stratified analysis exclusively (11), and by both approaches (33).

The extTADA methods calculates a Bayes factor (BF) and posterior probability of association (PPA) for each gene, and then converts PPA to FDR (false discovery rate) to identify candidate risk genes. Common FDR procedures are designed to control the proportion of false positives among discoveries. However, with a large number of known risk genes ranked among the top by PPA, the estimated FDR of novel genes will be smaller than their true values, considering the true FDR of known genes is 0. This will lead to inflation of the support for novel candidate genes (Kaplanis et al., 2020). To address this issue, we excluded 90 known genes with SFARI gene score 1 or 2 in FDR estimation (Supplementary Table 3.5). The stratified analysis yielded 71 candidate genes passing FDR ≤0.1, whereas unstratified analysis yielded 44 genes. Among these genes, 38 were identified exclusively by the stratified approach, 11 were exclusively found by the unstratified approach, and 33 were shared (Figure 3.8). Previous studies have shown that autism risk genes are often pleiotropic and implicated in other neurodevelopmental disorders (NDD) (Coe et al., 2019; Cross-Disorder Group of the Psychiatric Genomics Consortium. Electronic address & Cross-Disorder Group of the Psychiatric Genomics, 2019; Myers et al., 2020; Satterstrom et al., 2020). We obtained candidate NDD genes from a recent study(Kaplanis et al., 2020) to seek support of the candidate autism genes. Among the 38 genes identified only in stratified approach, 13 are significantly implicated with NDD. In contrast, only 1 out of the 11 unstratified-exclusive genes is implicated with NDD (Figure 3.9 and Supplementary table 3.6). Among the candidate genes

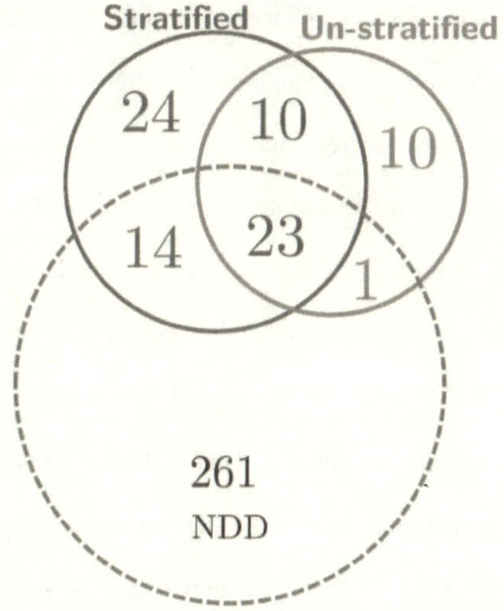

Figure 3.9 Additional support of candidate novel autism risk genes identified by stratified or unstratified extTADA analysis with significant genes in neurodevelopmental disorders (NDD) identified by Kaplanis et al 2020. Among 33 genes identified by both stratified and unstratified extTADA, 23 (70%) are implicated with NDD; 14 genes out of 38 (37%) identified exclusively by stratified extTADA are implicated with NDD, whereas only 1 out of 11 (9%) exclusively identified by unstratified extTADA is associated with NDD.

that are also implicated with NDD, several are notable with additional support from other studies on autism or syndromes with autistic features, such as *NR2F2, NR4A2, HNRNPU, CLCN4,* and *PRKAR1B* (Table 3.3). Candidate risk genes located in quadrant C, such as *GIGYF1* and *PRKAR1B*, are among the small number of candidate genes that are not constrained (pLI ~ 0).

3.2.4 Autism risk genes are highly expressed in deep-layer excitatory neurons in cortex

Previous studies have investigated autism risk by cortex laminar architecture. However, studies based on co-expression analysis (Parikshak et al., 2013; Willsey et al., 2013) or neurochemical experiments (Stoner et al., 2014; Trutzer, Garcia-Cabezas, & Zikopoulos, 2019) reported conflicting conclusions, that either deep or superficial layers of cortex are associated with autism. These early studies were based on a small number of high-confidence autism risk genes. Here we revisit the question with a much larger list of high-confidence candidate genes and single cell RNA-seq data. We obtained a single-nucleus RNA-seq data set of the middle temporal gyrus (MTG) of adult human cortex with clear laminar layer information (Hodge et al., 2019). The expression level of those 90 SFARI score 1 or 2 genes and 71 novel candidate risk genes is shown in the heatmap in Figure 3.10A. Hierarchical clustering based on the expression data forms four major clusters of genes. Genes in cluster 1 show very little expression in most cell types, except that *TBR1*, *RORB*, *MEIS2*, *PTCHD1*, *FEZF2* and *NR4A2* are sparsely expressed in subtypes excitatory neurons and *RELN* and *PCDH19* are highly expressed in subtypes of inhibitory neurons. Cluster 2 genes have more specific expression in deep-layer excitatory neurons. Genes in cluster 3 are expressed more widely in neuronal cell types with even higher expression in excitatory neurons at deep layers of MTG. Genes in cluster 4 have high expression in almost all the neuronal cell types in MTG. Mapping quadrant gene groups defined by A-risk and pLI into those 4 distinct expression clusters reveals that both cluster 3 and 4 are dominated by quadrant A genes (33 out of 47 genes and 29 out of 32 genes, respectively). Cluster 2 contains the largest portion of quadrant C genes (10 out of 16 genes, Figure 3.10B). Consistent with pLI value distribution, a larger fraction of genes in cluster 2 have higher observed to expected (O/E) ratio of LoF mutations in gnomAD (genome aggregation database)(Karczewski et al., 2020) compared to genes in other clusters (Figure 3.10C). Overall, excitatory neurons project from or to deep layers have high expression of the largest subset of known and candidate risk genes.

The heatmap of expression fraction in the same order of genes using the two fetal data sets in our model are shown in Figure 3.11. There is no layer information with the fetal data. Nevertheless, the expression patterns of candidate risk genes in the two fetal data sets generally follows the organization in the adult cortex data, especially for fetal prefrontal cortex. Additionally, 14 out of 24 cluster 1 genes with little expression in adult cortex neuronal cells have fraction expression ≥ 0.5 in at least one cell type in fetal prefrontal cortex, suggesting a dynamic temporal specific expression of those candidate risk genes.

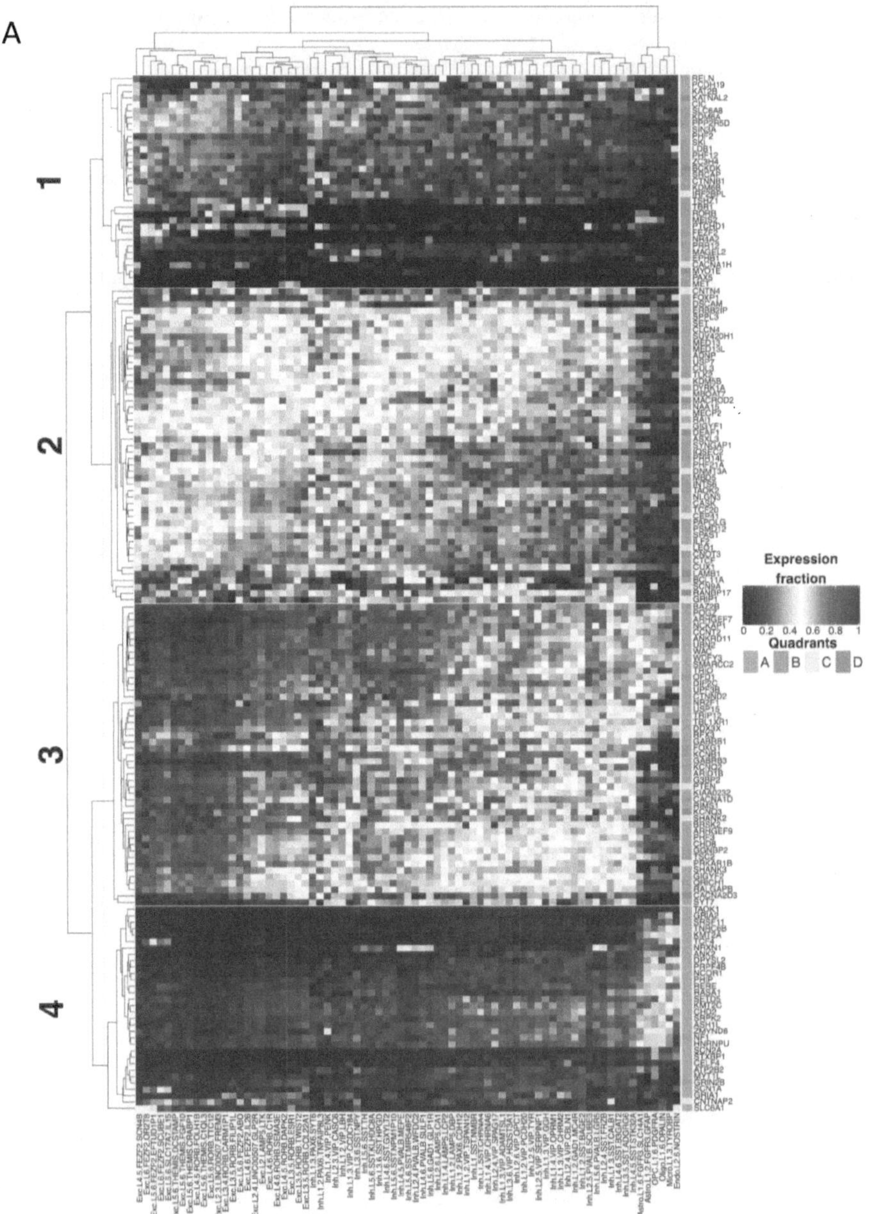

A
1
2
3
4
Expression fraction
0 0.2 0.4 0.6 0.8 1
Quadrants
A B C D

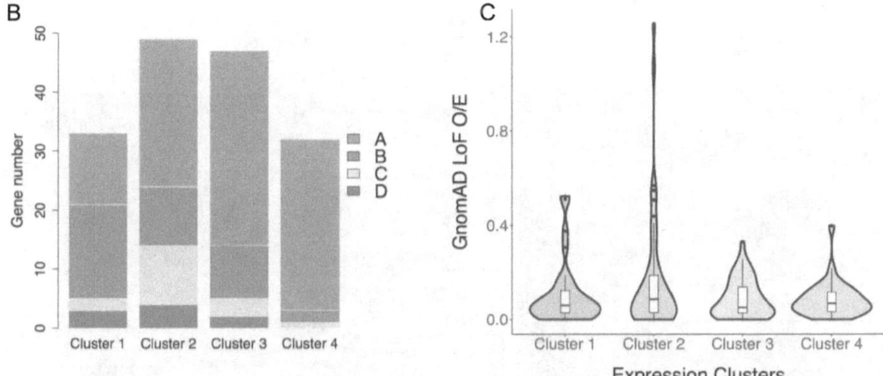

Figure 3.10 Most autism risk genes have high expression in deep-layer excitatory neurons in prefrontal cortex. (A) Hierarchical clustering 90 known autism risk genes and 71 novel candidate genes by expression level in cell types from adult cortex middle temporal gyrus (MTG) with laminar information. Genes (shown in rows) form 4 major clusters, labeled from 1 to 4 on the left. The dash line marks the height cutting the hierarchical tree. Cell types are clustered as well and are labels in the format as "major cell type.located layers.marker genes". Exc, excitatory neurons. Inh, inhibitory neurons. Astro, astrocytes. OPC, oligodendrocyte precursor cells. Oligo, oligodendrocytes. Micro, microglia. Endo, endothelial cells. The color (blue to red) of the heatmap indicates expression level of a gene in the cell type, calculated as the fraction of cells that have ≥1 UMI mapped to the gene in the cell type. Almost all genes in cluster 1 have low expression in all cell types. Most genes in cluster 2 are specifically expressed in excitatory neurons in deep layers (layer 4 to 6). Cluster 3 genes are highly expressed in deep excitatory neurons and have expression in most of neuronal cell types. Cluster 4 genes are highly expressed in almost all neuronal cell types. Quadrant gene groups stratified by Frisk and pLI are labeled by the color bar on the right side with A, B, C and D represented by orange, purple, yellow and green. (B) Number of known or candidate risk genes from quadrant gene groups in each expression clusters. Cluster 1 is enriched with quadrant B genes (high pLI and low A-risk); cluster 2 is enriched with quadrant C genes (low pLI and high A-risk); cluster 3 and 4 are enriched with quadrant A genes (high pLI and high A-risk). (C) The distribution of observed over expected (O/E) number of loss of function variants in gnomAD database in the 4 expression clusters. Cluster 2 genes have a broad distribution of O/E. Genes in other clusters have generally small O/E.

3.3 Discussion

In this study, we developed a new method, "A-risk", to predict plausibility of autism risk genes based on single-cell expression patterns in human fetal midbrain and prefrontal cortex. A-risk was trained using known autism genes. A-risk score reflects the similarity of the cell-type-specific expression pattern of a gene to known autism genes in aggregation. It achieves superior performance in prioritizing *de novo* risk variants, especially in genes that are less intolerant of

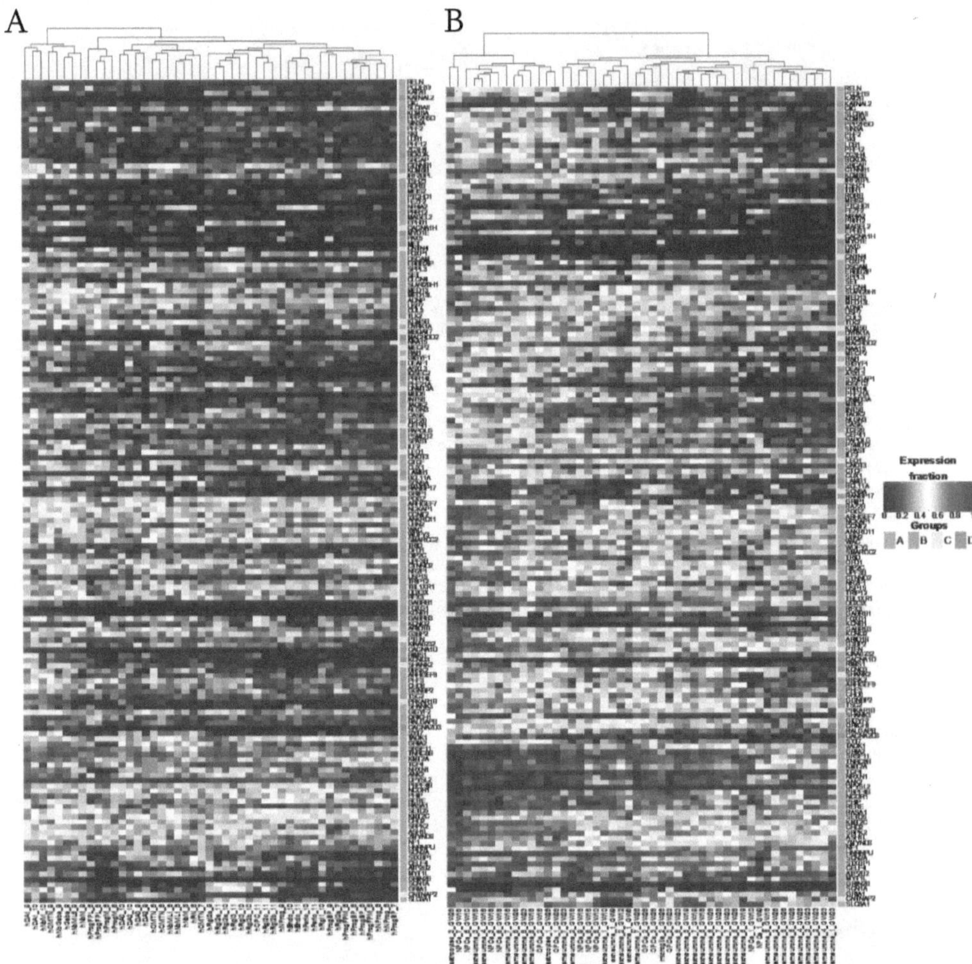

Figure 3.11 Heatmap of expression level of known and candidate risk genes in fetal midbrain (A) and prefrontal cortex (B). Row orders are arranged as same as Figure 3.8. Cell types in midbrain are labeled as "h(human)cell type names_week" and cell types in prefrontal cortex are labeled as "major cell type name_sub clusters_gestational weeks", in concordance with original data. DA, dopaminergic neurons. NbM, medial neuroblast. OMTN, oculomotor and trochlear nucleus. NbGaba, neuroblast GABAergic. Gaba, GABAergic neurons. NbML, mediolateral neuroblasts. ProgFPL, progenitor lateral floorplate. ProgM, progenitor midline. RN, red nucleus. Rgl, radial glia-like cells. OPC, oligodendrocyte precursor cells. NProg, neuronal progenitor. Endo, endothelial cells. Peric, pericytes. ProgBP, progenitor basal plate. ProgFPM, progenitor medial floorplate. NPCs, neural progenitor cells. Exneurons, excitatory neurons.

loss of function variants. Furthermore, A-risk is complementary with gene constraint metric (pLI) for improving estimation of priors using an empirical Bayesian association method. Applying it to published *de novo* variant data, we identified 71 novel candidate risk genes, an increase of 27 genes over the results using the same statistical method without stratification of genes by either A-risk or pLI.

Both inhibitory and excitatory neurons in the prefrontal cortex strongly contribute to A-risk prediction during fetal stages, consistent with previous theory of excitatory and inhibitory imbalance in the prefrontal cortex disrupting neural communication(Rubenstein, 2011; Zikopoulos & Barbas, 2013). GABAergic inhibitory neurons in midbrain have been identified as the most significant contributing feature to A-risk prediction, implicating a potential role of midbrain in autism pathogenesis that has been understudied.

Early functional and co-expression network studies (Chang et al., 2015; Willsey et al., 2013) based on a small number of high-confidence autism risk genes have revealed convergence on excitatory neurons in deep-cortical layers, however, another co-expression network analysis (Parikshak et al., 2013) found significance in excitatory neurons in superficial cortical layers. With a much larger number of high-confidence risk genes, we revisited the role of neuronal cell types in six different cortical layers. Based on a large single nuclei RNA-seq data set from adult cortex, we observed that deep-layer excitatory neurons have high expression of the vast majority of known and candidate autism risk genes, while other neuronal types or neurons in superficial layers have high expression of a much smaller subset of these genes. Since the excitatory neurons residing in layer 5 or 6 of cortex extend their axons into other regions of brain and communicate between cortex and other critical regions (Molyneaux, Arlotta, Menezes, & Macklis, 2007; Rubenstein, 2011), disruption of deep-layer excitatory neurons more likely affects signal transmission and communication across different brain regions. Taking account of gene mutation intolerance (pLI) and expression similarity to known autism genes (A-risk), the candidate risk genes with high A-risk but low pLI (i.e. quadrant C), such as *GIGYF1* and *MBOAT7,* are much more likely to have specific expression in deep-layer excitatory neurons. Interestingly, a recent study (Satterstrom et al.) showed *GIGYF1* was the most autism-specific gene among all candidate autism risk genes based on frequency of disruptive *de novo* variants in either autistic or severe NDD cohorts. This suggests an association of deep-layer excitatory neurons and autistic conditions that do not involve severe NDD conditions such as intellectual disabilities. We expect that this hypothesis will be tested in future studies with independent high-resolution single cells or neural circuit expression data, larger set of high-confidence risk genes, and autism cohorts with comprehensive NDD phenotyping.

The majority of genes in quadrant C are located in expression cluster 2, where a higher proportion of genes shows increased observed to expected (O/E) ratio of LoF mutations, suggesting quadrant C genes are less intolerant to LoF mutations or may be incompletely penetrant. The genes that have high A-risk and high pLI (quadrant A) are more likely to have high expression in a wide range of cell types. Candidate risk genes in cluster 1, among which 16 genes out of 33 in total have high pLI but low A-risk (quadrant B), have sparse expression in adult cortex but more expression in fetal prefrontal cortex, indicating those autism risk genes can take effect at limited time points and places.

A-risk directly utilized single-cell transcriptomic data as the input of the machine learning model to learn expression patterns from known risk genes. Expression patterns inferred from single-cell RNA-seq data have better resolution than bulk sequencing data with fine-grained cell-type heterogeneity and developmental temporal information. To integrate transcriptomic information in risk gene discovery in a principled way, we used A-risk in an empirical Bayesian framework to improve prior estimation based on genetic data. This approach yielded 27 more candidate risk genes than the original Bayesian approach using only genetic data. With increased sample sizes in the future, A-risk can also be used as informative covariates to improve FDR estimation (Ignatiadis, Klaus, Zaugg, & Huber; M. J. Zhang, Xia, & Zou) in frequentist approaches for risk gene discovery.

A-risk is currently limited by the availability of comprehensive single-cell expression profiles across all critical human brain regions and developmental stages. Profiling neuron cells is uniquely challenging since the information in extended projections and axons can be lost during sample preparation in single-cell RNA-seq. Even though the data we used in the A-risk model is from fetal stages, when extended axons of neurons have not been prolonged, we should still interpret with consideration that there could be some genes missed in the data. New single-nucleus RNA-seq and subcellular transcriptomic profiling techniques and data sets from ongoing projects such as Allen Brain Institutes (Miller et al., 2014) and Human Cell Atlas (Han et al., 2020) will help to address this issue (Fazal et al., 2019; Kebschull et al., 2016). Additionally, A-risk is a supervised learning approach, and inevitably it biases towards genes with similar expression patterns to known risk genes in the training. Unsupervised approaches could assist in addressing the problem. Finally, abundant and specific expression is not sufficient to define a gene as a risk gene. Other factors such as functional redundancy (Kafri, Levy, & Pilpel, 2006) and protein complex formation (Marianayagam, Sunde, & Matthews, 2004) that determine whether a high-expression gene is a bottleneck in a system, also play a role in the genetic impact. Future studies can consider those factors with single-cell expression profiles to improve accuracy of prediction.

3.4 Material and methods

3.4.1 Data collection and preprocessing

In this study, we integrated human fetal brain single-cell RNA-seq data from two publications: (1) midbrains from 6 to 11 weeks (La Manno et al., 2016) and (2) prefrontal cortexes from gestational weeks 8 to 26(Zhong et al., 2018). To integrate these two data sets, first, we obtained the UMI counts of single cells from their published data. Second, we directly utilized the cell type clusters and time points documented in the publications and calculated the expression fraction of each gene in each cell type at a particular time point. We combined each individual cell type and time point together to generalize one feature in the integrated data. The expression fraction is defined as, for a particular gene in a cell type at a developmental time point, the number of cells having the gene expressed (UMI >= 1) divided by the total number of cells grouped in the cell type. *La Manno et al., 2016*(La Manno et al., 2016) reported 26 cell types across 6 developmental time points, including an unknown cell type ("Unk") where those cells cannot be assigned to any known clusters. We excluded Unk cells in the analysis. *Zhong et al., 2018* reported clustered 35 cell types through 9 time points. Furthermore, we also excluded cell types with fewer than or equal to 10 cells. In total, we compiled 95 features in the combined data set, including 47 from *La Manno et al., 2016* and 48 features from *Zhong et al., 2018*.

We obtained known autism risk genes with score of 1 or 2 in the SFARI database(Abrahams et al., 2013) version released on 08/29/2019) as the positives for model training. There are 3 genes *BAZ2B*, *MSNP1AS* and *TBR1* not present in the single-cell expression data, so we excluded them in the positive training set. For the negatives for model training, we collected genes harboring at least 1 *de novo* LGD variant in controls from an exome-sequencing study on autism(Iossifov et al., 2014). Two genes (*KDM5B* and *CACNA1H*) are present in both the initial positive and negative sets. We removed these 2 genes from the negative set. In total, we compiled 88 genes in the positive training data set and 154 genes in the negative training data set. The full list of training genes is available in Supplementary table 3.1.

3.4.2 Machine learning approaches to predict autism risk genes

A-risk ("Autism risk") is based on a supervised machine-learning method, gradient boosting tree (GBT) (Friedman, 2002). The goal of the model is to find a function $F^*(x)$ mapping "input" x to "output" y, such that the expected value of some specified loss function $\Psi(y, F(x))$ is minimized,

$$F^*(x) = arg \min_{F(x)} Ey,x\, \Psi(y, F(x)).$$

GBT is estimating $F^*(x)$ by an additive update to the form

$$F(x) = \sum_{m=0}^{M} \beta_m h(x),$$

and specifically updating the previous model with the error estimated in the previous step

$$F_m(x) = F_{m-1}(x) + \beta_m h(x),$$

where the functions $h(x)$ are base learner functions and $m = 1,2,...,M$ is iteration of the model. β_m is the current "pseudo"-residual, where

$$\beta_{im} = -\frac{\partial \Psi(y, F_{m-1}(x))}{\partial F_{m-1}(x)} |x = x_i, y = y_i,$$

for all $i = 1,2,...,N$, which is the number of training data points. Then we can estimate the optimal β_m and base learner $h(x)$ by fitting

$$\beta_m = \text{arg} \min_{\beta} \sum_{i=1}^{N} \Psi(y_i, F_{m-1}(x_i) + \beta h(x)).$$

We train the model using the training gene set and features derived from single cell data sets. To implement the gradient boosting tree machine, we used the python package "sklearn.ensemble.GradientBoostingClassifier" with parameters of "n_estimators" as 300, "learning_rate" as 0.05 and "max_depth" as 1. We assessed the performance of the model by 5-fold cross validation. In each cross validation, the model randomly selected 20% of the training gene set to serve as a test set for validation and the rest of the genes were used to train the model. We implemented the python package "sklearn.metrics.roc_curve" to calculate the true positive rate, false positive rate, and to plot the ROC curve and calculate AUC values. After training, we predicted the probability for each protein-coding gene in the genome being a positive gene (i.e. plausibility for being an autism risk gene) by the trained model. The final A-risk score is the average probability from the 5-fold training and prediction. The complete A-risk score is available in Supplementary table 2.

"Feature importance" is derived from the gradient boosting tree model using the function "feature_importances_". In the GBT model, parameters of base learner functions are the splitting variables and corresponding split points defining the tree. The "feature_importances_" is a normalized estimate of the predictive power of a particular feature by combining the fraction of samples the feature contributes to and the decrease in impurity from splitting them (Louppe, 2014). The final feature importance value for each selected feature is the average from the 5-fold training and prediction. All selected features with non-zero feature importance are listed in Supplementary table 2.

3.4.3 Comparison of A-risk to other metrices in prioritizing *de novo* LGD variants

We tool two approaches to compare the ability of A-risk and other metrics in prioritization of *de novo* variants. With each metric, we first rank all genes; then in all genes above a certain rank threshold (e.g. 1000, 1500, 2000, etc), we estimated the "enrichment of *de novo* variants", "precision", and "true positives". The formulae to compute these estimates are as following:

For any gene $\boldsymbol{i}$, the number of expected *de novo* variants in each gene, $\boldsymbol{E_i}$, was calculated as:

$$\boldsymbol{E_i = 2 \times N \times r_i}$$

where $\boldsymbol{N}$ is the number of trios in the compiled data sets and $\boldsymbol{r_i}$ is gene-specific background mutation rate. Here we tested on *de novo* gene-likely disrupting (LGD) variants and deleterious missense (D-mis) variants (Figure 3.4). LGD variants include nonsense, frameshift and canonical splice site mutations and D-mis variants are defined as variants with REVEL (the Rare Exome Variant Ensemble Learner) score >= 0.5 (Ioannidis et al., 2016). For each gene, $\boldsymbol{r_i}$ is the sum of background mutation rate of LGD mutations plus D-mis mutations.

The background mutation rate per gene of each mutation type was obtained from a previous described mutation model (Carlson et al., 2018; Samocha et al., 2014). Briefly, the seven-nucleotide sequence context was used to determine the probability of each base in mutating to each other possible base. Then, the mutation rate of each functional class in each gene was calculated by adding up point mutation rates in the longest transcript. The rate of frameshift indels was presumed to be 1.25 times the nonsense mutation rate and the rate of genes located on chromosome X is further adjusted according to female-to-male ratio in the *de novo* data set (C. F. Wright et al., 2015).

For a set of genes, the enrichment of *de novo* variants, $\boldsymbol{D}$, was calculated as:

$$\boldsymbol{D} = \frac{\boldsymbol{M}}{\sum_i \boldsymbol{E}_i}$$

where $\boldsymbol{M}$ is the total number of observed *de novo* LGD or D-mis variants in this gene set. In this study, we compiled results from multiple whole exome studies on autism spectrum disorders, including total of 8838 trios from Simons Simplex Collection (SSC) (Iossifov et al., 2014), Autism Sequencing Consortium (ASC) (Satterstrom et al., 2020), SPARK Pilot (Feliciano et al., 2019), MSSNG (Yuen et al., 2017), Takata et al., 2018 (Takata et al., 2018) and Chen et al., 2017 (R. Chen et al., 2017) cohorts.

For any gene set, the number of detected true positives, $\boldsymbol{TP}$, was calculated as:

$$\boldsymbol{TP} = \boldsymbol{M} - \sum_i \boldsymbol{E}_i$$

For any gene set, the precision (positive predictive value), $\boldsymbol{PPV}$, was calculated as:

$$\boldsymbol{PPV} = \frac{M - \sum_i E_i}{M}$$

For each metric (A-risk, pLI etc.), a set of genes were selected based on the rank of genes by each individual metric, such as top 1000 genes or top 2000 genes, etc. The genome baseline is defined by all the genes in the genome. For the first estimate, enrichment of *de novo* variants, $\boldsymbol{D}$, was calculated for any set of top-ranked genes, and then enrichment values were plotted and compared, as shown in Figure 3.4A. For the second estimate, the number of detected true positives, $\boldsymbol{TP}$, and the precision (true discovery rate), $\boldsymbol{PPV}$, were calculated for any set of top-ranked genes. $\boldsymbol{TP}$ and $\boldsymbol{PPV}$ were plotted and compared, as shown in Figure 3.4B. Recall would be calculated as $R = \boldsymbol{TP}/N$, where N is the total number of true positives (N). Since N is unknown but a constant, $\boldsymbol{TP}$ is proportional to R. Therefore, we use TP as a proxy of recall. To avoid inflation of A-risk performance, we excluded all the known autism risk genes used in A-risk training during calculation of all above estimates. Although there are different numbers of genes predicted by each method, we compared all the methods with 18663 protein-coding genes, replacing missing scores with the median of each corresponding metrices.

To exam the potential of A-risk in prioritizing *de novo* variants in non-constrained genes, we limit the estimates on genes with pLI score <= 0.9 in each top rank of genes (Figure 3.5C and D). We excluded pLI as a metric for comparison in those figures since pLI was used to stratify constraint and non-constraint genes. Furthermore, we also compare A-risk with the other two metrices D-score and Krishnan 2016 (Figure 3.6).

3.4.4 Application of A-risk in stratified risk-gene discovery analysis

In this analysis, we used an empirical Bayesian model of rare-variant genetic architecture, extTADA (Extended Transmission and *de novo* Association) (Nguyen et al., 2017), which can estimate mean effect sizes and risk-gene proportions from the genetic data to identify autism candidate risk genes. The extTADA model is developed based on a previous integrated empirical Bayesian model TADA (Transmission and *de novo* Association) (X. He et al., 2013), but it advanced the framework by estimating parameters using MCMC (Markov Chain Monte Carlo) process so that more accurate estimation on local gene groups can be achieved and confidence intervals can be provided.

Two major parameters, relative risk of a gene causing a disease $\boldsymbol{\gamma}$ and the proportion of disease risk genes across the local gene groups $\boldsymbol{\pi}$, are estimated by the connection to variant fold enrichment (***FE***), which is calculated as the number of observed variants divided by the number of expected. Assuming the background mutation rate for each gene is $\boldsymbol{\mu}$, total number of genes in the gene set is $\boldsymbol{m}$ and total number of sequenced samples is $\boldsymbol{N}$, then

$$\text{the observed variants, } \boldsymbol{X = \pi m \times 2\gamma\mu N + (1\text{-}\pi) m \times 2\mu N}$$

the expected variants, $X_e = \pi m \times 2\mu N + (1-\pi) m \times 2\mu N$

$$FE = \frac{X}{Xe} = \pi(\gamma - 1) + 1,\ \gamma \sim Gamma\ (\bar{\gamma}\beta, \beta)$$

FE can be calculated from the data, parameters γ, π and β are estimated accordingly using a Hamiltonian Monte Carlo (HMC) MCMC method implemented in the "rstan" package (Carpenter et al., 2017).

Bayes factors can be estimated as following:

$$B = \frac{P(X|H1)}{P(X|H0)} \sim \frac{Pois(2\gamma\mu N)}{Pois(2\mu N)}$$

***H*1** is alternative hypothesis and ***H*0** is null, where $\gamma = 1$.

From Bayes' theorem, the posterior odds are equal to the Bayes factor times the prior odds:

$$\frac{P(H1|X)}{P(H0|X)} = \frac{P(X|H1)}{P(X|H0)} \times \frac{P(H1)}{P(H0)}$$

where $P(H1)$ is estimated π, $P(H0)$ is $(1-\pi)$.

Assuming the posterior probability of association (PPA), $P(H1|X)$ is q, so the posterior probability of the null model $P(H0|X)$ is $q_0 = (1 - q)$,

$$q = \frac{B\pi}{1-\pi+B\pi}$$

then per-gene based FDR can be calculated from q_0. First, q_0 is ranked in an increasing order for all the genes, then FDR is the sum of total q_0 smaller than the current rank @*k* divided by the total number of genes *k* with smaller q_0:

$$FDR@k = \frac{\sum_{k}^{i=1} q_{0i}}{k}$$

To inform the parameter estimation with prior knowledge, we stratify the whole genome into 4 quadrants by A-risk score 0.4 and pLI score 0.9, so extTADA can estimate local parameters in each 4 groups and better characterize properties for individual groups. Specifically, quadrant A consists of genes with A-risk >=0.4 and pLI >=0.9. Genes in quadrant B are in A-risk <0.4 but pLI >=0.9. Genes in quadrant C have A-risk >=0.4 but pLI <0.9, and the rest of the genes are assigned to quadrant D. We applied the extTADA model to each quadrant of genes to estimate the parameters and calculate PPAs. Then we combined the PPAs of 4 quadrants together to calculate a final genome-wide FDR (false discovery rate). To make FDR estimation of novel risk genes more accurate, we excluded known autism risk genes used in training A-risk model in FDR calculation, as most of these genes are ranked in top by PPA and including them in FDR calculation with deflate FDR values of novel risk genes. In parallel, we also inputted all genes into extTADA without stratification by A-risk or pLI to obtain an unstratified version of the same analysis, so that we can show the advantage of integration of biological information in genetic association studies. We used the same *de novo* variant data from 8838 trios and background mutation rate data as described above.

3.4.5 Expression pattern clustering of known and candidate autism risk genes

We compiled the 71 novel candidate risk genes that pass FDR <=0.1 in stratified extTADA analysis together with 90 known risk genes (The gene *MSNP1AS* is missing in the input data for extTADA, because it is a non-coding gene.) and investigated the expression pattern of all those risk genes in a single-cell RNA-seq data of adult human cortex (Hodge et al., 2019). The data was pre-processed as described above and the expression fraction for each cell type was pre-computed from read-count data downloaded from the publication. Hierarchical clustering was performed using "ComplexHeatmap" package in R based on "Euclidean distance" and the heatmap (Figure 3.10A) was drawn by the "heatmap" function built in the package.

Chapter 4: Conclusion and Discussion

4.1 Conclusion

This thesis discussed about two methods, *Episcore* and *A-risk*. The methods are built on data mining on functional genomics using machine learning approaches. *Episcore* has successfully predicted haploinsufficient genes by learning on analogous epigenomic patterns present in known haploinsufficient genes, such as broader peaks of H3K4me3 epigenomic modification and more frequent interactions between promoters and enhancers. We compiled about 360 features from various epigenomic modification in multiple human tissues or cell lines. By using *Episcore*, we can identify disease risk genes that take action through haploinsufficiency, which is the major mechanism when mutations occurred in risk genes. *A-risk* is a method developed specific to autism, where we learned from the single-cell expression patterns of known autism risk genes, and predicted on other genes vulnerable to autism genetic risks. We integrated two single-cell RNA-seq data sets from human fetal midbrain and prefrontal cortex, consisting about 4000 cells in a wide range of developmental stages. *A-risk* prioritized about 2500 genes and there is a significant enrichment of *de novo* LGD and deleterious missense mutations from autism patients among the top 2500 genes.

The two methods developed from functional genomics provide additional and orthogonal information for traditional genetic analysis, combining which gained improved power to identify and better interpret genetic risks. The most-adapted pLI metric is developed by measuring depletion of LoF mutations in healthy populations and only utilized WES data. By combining *Episcore* and pLI, the meta score can improve the precision and true positives to much higher levels, indicating the two methods are complementary and providing diverse biological information. The advantage of plugging *A-risk* into discovery of autism risk genes is even more prominent. After inputting A-risk as prior information for parameter estimation in extTADA analysis, we identified 27 more risk genes resulting in total of 71 novel risk genes except for all known risk genes, with current limited sample size.

Data mining on functional genomics can directing infer disease etiology. The common obstacles of genetic analysis lie in lack of linkage to functional interpretation, so when we found a risk gene with strong statistic evidence, it is hard to find mode of action and implicated cell types, tissue or developmental time point. In both Episcore and A-risk, we predict on risk genes directly from their regulatory or transcriptomic landscapes, therefore we can interpret disease mechanism altogether. In Episcore, the importance directly derived from the random forest model shows that active promoters and enhancers have more contribution to haploinsufficiency than repressive promoter features, indicating regulations for haploinsufficient genes may come from active promoters and enhancers more. Similarly, we also inferred from the A-risk model that GABAergic neurons at week 9 in midbrain and excitatory neurons at week 12 in prefrontal cortex are the most contributing cell types to autism risk prediction, which means that those may be the most vulnerable cell types in autism etiology providing directions for future functional studies. In summary, we found that integrating functional genomic data with genetic analysis is effective and tantalizing in facilitating genetic discoveries in era of computational biology.

In the following section, I am going to talk about future steps to improve our prediction models and methods. In addition, I am going to propose other directions to integrate functional data into genetic studies.

4.2 Discussion

4.2.1 Transmission risk analysis in A-risk gene discovery

Even though A-risk autism genes are predicted by training on risk genes identified by *de novo* variants, we still interested in how A-risk risk genes can characterize autism genetic architecture. A current ongoing analysis working on the SPARK (Simons Powering Autism Research) project, which consist of WES data from more than 10,000 autism cases from about 9,000 families, analyzed the over-transmission rare LoF variants in multiple functional gene sets to compare for the most efficient metrics to prioritize rare inherited variants. They have compared between the number of transmitted and un-transmitted rare LoF variants from parents to affected offspring. The background gene set is composed of genes with pLI score > 0.5 as preliminary filtering and they selected several functional gene groups beyond it. A-risk candidate genes are selected by predicted score > 0.4 and are compared to the following gene sets: (1) Brain enriched genes are a specific group based on a transcriptome analysis, that expressed in brain tissues with larger than 5 times median expression in other tissues (Fagerberg et al., 2014). (2) SynaptomeDB is a database collecting proteome comprising the synaptome (Pirooznia et al., 2012), a critical implicated regulome in autism. (3) FMRP interacts with transcripts encoding pre- and postsynaptic proteins implicated in autism, so target genes of FMRP are potential convergent regulome for autism risks (Darnell et al., 2011). (4) Target genes of the autism-associated chromatin modifier CHD8 are also enriched for other ASD risk genes and converge in ASD-associated co-expression networks in human midfetal cortex (Cotney et al., 2015). (5) Targets of CELF4 are also enriched in the processes regulating synaptic plasticity and transmission (Wagnon et al., 2012). (6) The LOEUF metric stands for the "loss-of-function observed/expected upper bound fraction", which also measures the intolerance of a gene to variants but provides better significance measure than pLI (Karczewski et al., 2020). In this analysis, they found that A-risk explains the highest proportion (~60%) of over-transmitted events across all other 6 gene groups and achieves the highest precision as well, indicating A-risk candidate gene set performs best in prioritizing rare inherited LoF variants.

Following the same logic, we can also investigate the enrichment of common risk variants in A-risk candidate genes. Since A-risk genes are predicted on expression patterns of genes identified by *de novo* variants, higher enrichment of over transmission in A-risk predicted autism genes suggests inherited and de novo genetic risks can converge on common transcriptomic network or pathways in affected cell types. To further modify A-risk model to investigate the role of rare inherited variants, we can exclude positive training genes with nearly complete penetrance to train the machine learning model and find more risk genes vulnerable to inherited variants and identify implicated cell types.

4.2.2 The integration of more comprehensive data sets

The capacity of *Episcore* can be definitely improved by the availability of cell-type specific epigenomic data. A recent study using single-cell ATAC-seq (Assay for Transposase-Accessible Chromatin using sequencing) technique has profiled chromatin accessibility of >75,000 single cells from eight distinct arears of developing human forebrain (Ziffra et al., 2020), and the data can be adapted in *Episcore* model to gain more insights on regulatory mechanism on gene expression in the resolution of cell types of developing human brain. Their finding also showed the important contribution of specific and dynamic chromatin state to emerging cell-type diversity and cell fate specification, indicating additional cell-type epigenomic information can be leveraged by *Episcore* model. Furthermore, cell-type epigenomics of mouse cerebrum have been profiled as well (Li et al., 2020), which we can also integrate in the model to better understand mammalian brain regulation.

In the meantime, another straight forward direction to improve *A-risk* method is to compile and integrate more single-cell transcriptomic data. First, data from other tissues or areas of human brain can be combined to investigate genetic risk impact in other brain structures, for example, spatial and single-cell data from striatum (Martin et al., 2019) and cerebellum (Aldinger et al., 2020). Second, we can collect data from other important developmental stages. In our original *A-risk* model, we didn't include a considerable number of neuronal cells during early second trimester stage, but a recent study has sequenced on 40,000 cells in human neocortex during mi-gestation (Polioudakis et al., 2019), with which can help complete the time-point gap in the previous *A-risk* model. We also believe that with more data collected in consortium projects like Allen Brain Map (Miller et al., 2014), the whole picture of human brain transcriptomics can be accessible in the near future.

Besides to improve the two methods we have developed, the machine-learning approach to predict on genetic risks can be applied to other diseases. There are aggregative studies profiling comprehensive transcriptomics across all major human organs to build a human cell landscape at single-cell level (Han et al., 2020; S. He et al., 2020). Consortiums like Human Cell Atlas (HCA, https://www.humancellatlas.org) has also been working on constructing systematic, high-resolution and comprehensive reference maps for all human cells. With more accessible data, the framework of *Episcore* or *A-risk* can be applied to facilitate risk gene discovery and extend our understanding in other diseases.

4.2.3 Single-cell RNA velocity Analysis on transcriptional regulation of disease risk genes

A recent study brought up a concept, RNA velocity γ in single cells, to measure cellular dynamics using single-cell RNA-seq data (La Manno et al., 2018)(La Manno, 2018). Assuming a steady-state abundance of spliced (mature) s and unspliced (nascent) u mRNA molecules captured by single-cell RNA-seq technique, this method estimates RNA velocity of a particular gene from the snap-shot of expression (t indicates time):

$$\frac{ds}{dt} = u - \gamma s$$

Where γ is a composite value combining degradation and splicing rates and capturing gene and cell-type specific regulatory properties, which can be used as transcriptional dynamic measurements and cellular lineage indicators.

In *Episcore* and *A-risk,* we analyzed the epigenomic and expression pattern of risk genes. Higher level of expression or more sophisticated epigenomic regulation that a gene possesses is indeed an indicator of functional importance of the gene, but the regulatory dynamics is not inferred or leveraged in the model. By combining RNA velocity data in our machine learning approach, we can take advantage of the cellular dynamic information to understand the trajectory of disease risk genes in cellular differentiation process and identify more informative cell types shaping the disease etiology. By analyzing the enrichment of disease risk genes among those "driver genes" inferred by RNA velocity, we can also find relevant cell types involved in the pathology of the disease and gain more insights into disease genes' functional regulation.

References

Abrahams, B. S., Arking, D. E., Campbell, D. B., Mefford, H. C., Morrow, E. M., Weiss, L. A., . . . Packer, A. (2013). SFARI Gene 2.0: a community-driven knowledgebase for the autism spectrum disorders (ASDs). *Mol Autism, 4*(1), 36. doi:10.1186/2040-2392-4-36

Akazawa, H., & Komuro, I. (2005). Cardiac transcription factor Csx/Nkx2-5: Its role in cardiac development and diseases. *Pharmacol Ther, 107*(2), 252-268. doi:10.1016/j.pharmthera.2005.03.005

Aldinger, K. A., Thomson, Z., Haldipur, P., Deng, M., Timms, A. E., Hirano, M., . . . Millen, K. J. (2020). Spatial and single-cell transcriptional landscape of human cerebellar development. *bioRxiv*, 2020.2006.2030.174391. doi:10.1101/2020.06.30.174391

Alkuraya, F. S., Saadi, I., Lund, J. J., Turbe-Doan, A., Morton, C. C., & Maas, R. L. (2006). SUMO1 haploinsufficiency leads to cleft lip and palate. *Science, 313*(5794), 1751. doi:10.1126/science.1128406

Amaral, D. G., Schumann, C. M., & Nordahl, C. W. (2008). Neuroanatomy of autism. *Trends Neurosci, 31*(3), 137-145. doi:10.1016/j.tins.2007.12.005

Bailey, A., Le Couteur, A., Gottesman, I., Bolton, P., Simonoff, E., Yuzda, E., & Rutter, M. (1995). Autism as a strongly genetic disorder: evidence from a British twin study. *Psychol Med, 25*(1), 63-77. doi:10.1017/s0033291700028099

Baio, J., Wiggins, L., Christensen, D. L., Maenner, M. J., Daniels, J., Warren, Z., . . . Dowling, N. F. (2018). Prevalence of Autism Spectrum Disorder Among Children Aged 8 Years - Autism and Developmental Disabilities Monitoring Network, 11 Sites, United States, 2014. *MMWR Surveill Summ, 67*(6), 1-23. doi:10.15585/mmwr.ss6706a1

Benayoun, B. A., Pollina, E. A., Ucar, D., Mahmoudi, S., Karra, K., Wong, E. D., . . . Brunet, A. (2014). H3K4me3 breadth is linked to cell identity and transcriptional consistency. *Cell, 158*(3), 673-688. doi:10.1016/j.cell.2014.06.027

Benson, D. W., Silberbach, G. M., Kavanaugh-McHugh, A., Cottrill, C., Zhang, Y., Riggs, S., . . . Kugler, J. D. (1999). Mutations in the cardiac transcription factor NKX2.5 affect diverse cardiac developmental pathways. *J Clin Invest, 104*(11), 1567-1573. doi:10.1172/JCI8154

Brown, S. A., Warburton, D., Brown, L. Y., Yu, C. Y., Roeder, E. R., Stengel-Rutkowski, S., . . . Muenke, M. (1998). Holoprosencephaly due to mutations in ZIC2, a homologue of Drosophila odd-paired. *Nat Genet, 20*(2), 180-183. doi:10.1038/2484

Brueggeman, L., Koomar, T., & Michaelson, J. J. (2018). Forecasting autism gene discovery with machine learning and genome-scale data. *bioRxiv*, 370601. doi:10.1101/370601

Cao, H., Alston, L., Ruschman, J., & Hegele, R. A. (2008). Heterozygous CAV1 frameshift mutations (MIM 601047) in patients with atypical partial lipodystrophy and hypertriglyceridemia. *Lipids Health Dis, 7*, 3. doi:10.1186/1476-511X-7-3

Cardarelli, L., Maxwell, K. L., & Davidson, A. R. (2011). Assembly mechanism is the key determinant of the dosage sensitivity of a phage structural protein. *Proceedings of the National Academy of Sciences, 108*(25), 10168-10173. doi:10.1073/pnas.1100759108

Carlson, J., Locke, A. E., Flickinger, M., Zawistowski, M., Levy, S., Myers, R. M., . . . Consortium, B. (2018). Extremely rare variants reveal patterns of germline mutation rate heterogeneity in humans. *Nat Commun, 9*(1), 3753. doi:10.1038/s41467-018-05936-5

Carpenter, B., Gelman, A., Hoffman, M. D., Lee, D., Goodrich, B., Betancourt, M., . . . Riddell, A. (2017). Stan: A Probabilistic Programming Language. *2017, 76*(1), 32. doi:10.18637/jss.v076.i01

Cassa, C. A., Weghorn, D., Balick, D. J., Jordan, D. M., Nusinow, D., Samocha, K. E., . . . Sunyaev, S. R. (2017). Estimating the selective effects of heterozygous protein-truncating variants from human exome data. *Nat Genet, 49*(5), 806-810. doi:10.1038/ng.3831

Chang, J., Gilman, S. R., Chiang, A. H., Sanders, S. J., & Vitkup, D. (2015). Genotype to phenotype relationships in autism spectrum disorders. *Nat Neurosci, 18*(2), 191-198. doi:10.1038/nn.3907

Chen, C. A., Bosch, D. G., Cho, M. T., Rosenfeld, J. A., Shinawi, M., Lewis, R. A., . . . Schaaf, C. (2016). The expanding clinical phenotype of Bosch-Boonstra-Schaaf optic atrophy syndrome: 20 new cases and possible genotype-phenotype correlations. *Genet Med, 18*(11), 1143-1150. doi:10.1038/gim.2016.18

Chen, K., Chen, Z., Wu, D., Zhang, L., Lin, X., Su, J., . . . Li, W. (2015a). Broad H3K4me3 is associated with increased transcription elongation and enhancer activity at tumor-suppressor genes. *Nat Genet, 47*(10), 1149-1157. doi:10.1038/ng.3385

Chen, K., Chen, Z., Wu, D., Zhang, L., Lin, X., Su, J., . . . Li, W. (2015b). Broad H3K4me3 is associated with increased transcription elongation and enhancer activity at tumor-suppressor genes. *Nat Genet*. doi:10.1038/ng.3385

Chen, M., David, C. J., & Manley, J. L. (2012). Concentration-dependent control of pyruvate kinase M mutually exclusive splicing by hnRNP proteins. *Nat Struct Mol Biol, 19*(3), 346-354. doi:10.1038/nsmb.2219

Chen, R., Davis, L. K., Guter, S., Wei, Q., Jacob, S., Potter, M. H., . . . Li, B. (2017). Leveraging blood serotonin as an endophenotype to identify de novo and rare variants involved in autism. *Mol Autism, 8*, 14. doi:10.1186/s13229-017-0130-3

Coe, B. P., Stessman, H. A. F., Sulovari, A., Geisheker, M. R., Bakken, T. E., Lake, A. M., . . . Eichler, E. E. (2019). Neurodevelopmental disease genes implicated by de novo mutation and copy number variation morbidity. *Nat Genet, 51*(1), 106-116. doi:10.1038/s41588-018-0288-4

Colantuoni, C., Lipska, B. K., Ye, T., Hyde, T. M., Tao, R., Leek, J. T., . . . Kleinman, J. E. (2011). Temporal dynamics and genetic control of transcription in the human prefrontal cortex. *Nature, 478*(7370), 519-523. doi:10.1038/nature10524

Consortium, E. P., Bernstein, B. E., Birney, E., Dunham, I., Green, E. D., Gunter, C., & Snyder, M. (2012). An integrated encyclopedia of DNA elements in the human genome. *Nature, 489*(7414), 57-74. doi:10.1038/nature11247

Constantino, J. N., Zhang, Y., Frazier, T., Abbacchi, A. M., & Law, P. (2010). Sibling recurrence and the genetic epidemiology of autism. *Am J Psychiatry, 167*(11), 1349-1356. doi:10.1176/appi.ajp.2010.09101470

Cotney, J., Muhle, R. A., Sanders, S. J., Liu, L., Willsey, A. J., Niu, W., . . . Noonan, J. P. (2015). The autism-associated chromatin modifier CHD8 regulates other autism risk genes during human neurodevelopment. *Nat Commun, 6*, 6404. doi:10.1038/ncomms7404

Cross-Disorder Group of the Psychiatric Genomics Consortium. Electronic address, p. m. h. e., & Cross-Disorder Group of the Psychiatric Genomics, C. (2019). Genomic Relationships,

Novel Loci, and Pleiotropic Mechanisms across Eight Psychiatric Disorders. *Cell, 179*(7), 1469-1482 e1411. doi:10.1016/j.cell.2019.11.020

D'Ardenne, K., Eshel, N., Luka, J., Lenartowicz, A., Nystrom, L. E., & Cohen, J. D. (2012). Role of prefrontal cortex and the midbrain dopamine system in working memory updating. *Proc Natl Acad Sci U S A, 109*(49), 19900-19909. doi:10.1073/pnas.1116727109

Dang, V. T., Kassahn, K. S., Marcos, A. E., & Ragan, M. A. (2008). Identification of human haploinsufficient genes and their genomic proximity to segmental duplications. *Eur J Hum Genet, 16*(11), 1350-1357. doi:10.1038/ejhg.2008.111

Darnell, J. C., Van Driesche, S. J., Zhang, C., Hung, K. Y., Mele, A., Fraser, C. E., . . . Darnell, R. B. (2011). FMRP stalls ribosomal translocation on mRNAs linked to synaptic function and autism. *Cell, 146*(2), 247-261. doi:10.1016/j.cell.2011.06.013

Davoli, T., Xu, A. W., Mengwasser, K. E., Sack, L. M., Yoon, J. C., Park, P. J., & Elledge, S. J. (2013). Cumulative haploinsufficiency and triplosensitivity drive aneuploidy patterns and shape the cancer genome. *Cell, 155*(4), 948-962. doi:10.1016/j.cell.2013.10.011

De Rubeis, S., He, X., Goldberg, A. P., Poultney, C. S., Samocha, K., Cicek, A. E., . . . Buxbaum, J. D. (2014). Synaptic, transcriptional and chromatin genes disrupted in autism. *Nature, 515*(7526), 209-215. doi:10.1038/nature13772

Deciphering Developmental Disorders, S. (2015). Large-scale discovery of novel genetic causes of developmental disorders. *Nature, 519*(7542), 223-228. doi:10.1038/nature14135

Dekker, J., Belmont, A. S., Guttman, M., Leshyk, V. O., Lis, J. T., Lomvardas, S., . . . Zhong, S. (2017). The 4D Nucleome Project. *bioRxiv*. Retrieved from http://biorxiv.org/content/early/2017/01/26/103499.abstract

Dixon, J. R., Selvaraj, S., Yue, F., Kim, A., Li, Y., Shen, Y., . . . Ren, B. (2012). Topological domains in mammalian genomes identified by analysis of chromatin interactions. *Nature, 485*(7398), 376-380. doi:10.1038/nature11082

Dupays, L., Shang, C., Wilson, R., Kotecha, S., Wood, S., Towers, N., & Mohun, T. (2015). Sequential Binding of MEIS1 and NKX2-5 on the Popdc2 Gene: A Mechanism for Spatiotemporal Regulation of Enhancers during Cardiogenesis. *Cell Rep, 13*(1), 183-195. doi:10.1016/j.celrep.2015.08.065

Fagerberg, L., Hallstrom, B. M., Oksvold, P., Kampf, C., Djureinovic, D., Odeberg, J., . . . Uhlen, M. (2014). Analysis of the human tissue-specific expression by genome-wide integration of transcriptomics and antibody-based proteomics. *Mol Cell Proteomics, 13*(2), 397-406. doi:10.1074/mcp.M113.035600

Fang, R., Yu, M., Li, G., Chee, S., Liu, T., Schmitt, A. D., & Ren, B. (2016). Mapping of long-range chromatin interactions by proximity ligation-assisted ChIP-seq. *Cell Res, 26*(12), 1345-1348. doi:10.1038/cr.2016.137

Fantes, J., Ragge, N. K., Lynch, S. A., McGill, N. I., Collin, J. R., Howard-Peebles, P. N., . . . FitzPatrick, D. R. (2003). Mutations in SOX2 cause anophthalmia. *Nat Genet, 33*(4), 461-463. doi:10.1038/ng1120

Fazal, F. M., Han, S., Parker, K. R., Kaewsapsak, P., Xu, J., Boettiger, A. N., . . . Ting, A. Y. (2019). Atlas of Subcellular RNA Localization Revealed by APEX-Seq. *Cell, 178*(2), 473-490 e426. doi:10.1016/j.cell.2019.05.027

Feliciano, P., Zhou, X., Astrovskaya, I., Turner, T. N., Wang, T., Brueggeman, L., . . . Chung, W. K. (2019). Exome sequencing of 457 autism families recruited online provides evidence for autism risk genes. *NPJ Genom Med, 4*, 19. doi:10.1038/s41525-019-0093-8

Friedman, J. H. (2002). Stochastic gradient boosting. *Computational Statistics & Data Analysis, 38*(4), 367-378. doi:https://doi.org/10.1016/S0167-9473(01)00065-2

Geschwind, D. H. (2011). Genetics of autism spectrum disorders. *Trends Cogn Sci, 15*(9), 409-416. doi:10.1016/j.tics.2011.07.003

Giannakou, A., Sicko, R. J., Zhang, W., Romitti, P., Browne, M. L., Caggana, M., . . . Mills, J. L. (2017). Copy number variants in Ebstein anomaly. *PLoS One, 12*(12), e0188168. doi:10.1371/journal.pone.0188168

Gilman, S. R., Iossifov, I., Levy, D., Ronemus, M., Wigler, M., & Vitkup, D. (2011). Rare de novo variants associated with autism implicate a large functional network of genes involved in formation and function of synapses. *Neuron, 70*(5), 898-907. doi:10.1016/j.neuron.2011.05.021

Gonzalez, A. J., Setty, M., & Leslie, C. S. (2015). Early enhancer establishment and regulatory locus complexity shape transcriptional programs in hematopoietic differentiation. *Nat Genet*. doi:10.1038/ng.3402

Hamdan, F. F., Srour, M., Capo-Chichi, J. M., Daoud, H., Nassif, C., Patry, L., . . . Michaud, J. L. (2014). De novo mutations in moderate or severe intellectual disability. *PLoS Genet, 10*(10), e1004772. doi:10.1371/journal.pgen.1004772

Han, X., Zhou, Z., Fei, L., Sun, H., Wang, R., Chen, Y., . . . Guo, G. (2020). Construction of a human cell landscape at single-cell level. *Nature*. doi:10.1038/s41586-020-2157-4

Hastie, N. D. (1992). Dominant negative mutations in the Wilms tumour (WT1) gene cause Denys-Drash syndrome--proof that a tumour-suppressor gene plays a crucial role in normal genitourinary development. *Hum Mol Genet, 1*(5), 293-295. Retrieved from https://www.ncbi.nlm.nih.gov/pubmed/1338905

He, S., Wang, L.-h., Liu, Y., Li, Y.-q., Chen, H., Xu, J., . . . Guo, Z. (2020). Single-cell transcriptome profiling an adult human cell atlas of 15 major organs. *bioRxiv*, 2020.2003.2018.996975. doi:10.1101/2020.03.18.996975

He, X., Sanders, S. J., Liu, L., De Rubeis, S., Lim, E. T., Sutcliffe, J. S., . . . Roeder, K. (2013). Integrated model of de novo and inherited genetic variants yields greater power to identify risk genes. *PLoS Genet, 9*(8), e1003671. doi:10.1371/journal.pgen.1003671

Hodge, R. D., Bakken, T. E., Miller, J. A., Smith, K. A., Barkan, E. R., Graybuck, L. T., . . . Lein, E. S. (2019). Conserved cell types with divergent features in human versus mouse cortex. *Nature, 573*(7772), 61-68. doi:10.1038/s41586-019-1506-7

Homsy, J., Zaidi, S., Shen, Y., Ware, J. S., Samocha, K. E., Karczewski, K. J., . . . Chung, W. K. (2015). De novo mutations in congenital heart disease with neurodevelopmental and other congenital anomalies. *Science, 350*(6265), 1262-1266. doi:10.1126/science.aac9396

Homsy, J., Zaidi, S., Shen, Y., Ware, J. S., Samocha, K. E., Karczewski, K. J., . . . Chung, W. K. (2015). De novo mutations in congenital heart disease with neurodevelopmental and other congenital anomalies. *Science, 350*(6265), 1262-1266. doi:10.1126/science.aac9396

Huang, N., Lee, I., Marcotte, E. M., & Hurles, M. E. (2010). Characterising and predicting haploinsufficiency in the human genome. *PLoS Genet, 6*(10), e1001154. doi:10.1371/journal.pgen.1001154

Ignatiadis, N., Klaus, B., Zaugg, J. B., & Huber, W. (2016). Data-driven hypothesis weighting increases detection power in genome-scale multiple testing. *Nat Methods*. doi:10.1038/nmeth.3885

Ioannidis, N. M., Rothstein, J. H., Pejaver, V., Middha, S., McDonnell, S. K., Baheti, S., . . . Sieh, W. (2016). REVEL: An Ensemble Method for Predicting the Pathogenicity of Rare Missense Variants. *Am J Hum Genet, 99*(4), 877-885. doi:10.1016/j.ajhg.2016.08.016

Iossifov, I., O'Roak, B. J., Sanders, S. J., Ronemus, M., Krumm, N., Levy, D., . . . Wigler, M. (2014). The contribution of de novo coding mutations to autism spectrum disorder. *Nature, 515*(7526), 216-221. doi:10.1038/nature13908
10.1038/nature13908. Epub 2014 Oct 29.

Irvine, G. B., El-Agnaf, O. M., Shankar, G. M., & Walsh, D. M. (2008). Protein aggregation in the brain: the molecular basis for Alzheimer's and Parkinson's diseases. *Mol Med, 14*(7-8), 451-464. doi:10.2119/2007-00100.Irvine

Jin, S. C., Homsy, J., Zaidi, S., Lu, Q., Morton, S., DePalma, S. R., . . . Brueckner, M. (2017). Contribution of rare inherited and de novo variants in 2,871 congenital heart disease probands. *Nat Genet.* doi:10.1038/ng.3970

Kafri, R., Levy, M., & Pilpel, Y. (2006). The regulatory utilization of genetic redundancy through responsive backup circuits. *Proc Natl Acad Sci U S A, 103*(31), 11653-11658. doi:10.1073/pnas.0604883103

Kaplanis, J., Samocha, K. E., Wiel, L., Zhang, Z., Arvai, K. J., Eberhardt, R. Y., . . . Retterer, K. (2020). Integrating healthcare and research genetic data empowers the discovery of 28 novel developmental disorders. *bioRxiv*.

Karayiorgou, M., Simon, T. J., & Gogos, J. A. (2010). 22q11.2 microdeletions: linking DNA structural variation to brain dysfunction and schizophrenia. *Nat Rev Neurosci, 11*(6), 402-416. doi:10.1038/nrn2841

Karczewski, K. J., Francioli, L. C., Tiao, G., Cummings, B. B., Alfoldi, J., Wang, Q., . . . MacArthur, D. G. (2020). The mutational constraint spectrum quantified from variation in 141,456 humans. *Nature, 581*(7809), 434-443. doi:10.1038/s41586-020-2308-7

Kebschull, J. M., Garcia da Silva, P., Reid, A. P., Peikon, I. D., Albeanu, D. F., & Zador, A. M. (2016). High-Throughput Mapping of Single-Neuron Projections by Sequencing of Barcoded RNA. *Neuron, 91*(5), 975-987. doi:10.1016/j.neuron.2016.07.036

Kinoshita, A., Saito, T., Tomita, H., Makita, Y., Yoshida, K., Ghadami, M., . . . Yoshiura, K. (2000). Domain-specific mutations in TGFB1 result in Camurati-Engelmann disease. *Nat Genet, 26*(1), 19-20. doi:10.1038/79128

Klein, A. M., & Treutlein, B. (2019). Single cell analyses of development in the modern era. *Development, 146*(12). doi:10.1242/dev.181396

Kodo, K., Nishizawa, T., Furutani, M., Arai, S., Yamamura, E., Joo, K., . . . Yamagishi, H. (2009). GATA6 mutations cause human cardiac outflow tract defects by disrupting semaphorin-plexin signaling. *Proc Natl Acad Sci U S A, 106*(33), 13933-13938. doi:10.1073/pnas.0904744106

Krishnan, A., Zhang, R., Yao, V., Theesfeld, C. L., Wong, A. K., Tadych, A., . . . Troyanskaya, O. G. (2016). Genome-wide prediction and functional characterization of the genetic basis of autism spectrum disorder. *Nat Neurosci, 19*(11), 1454-1462. doi:10.1038/nn.4353

Krumm, N., O'Roak, B. J., Shendure, J., & Eichler, E. E. (2014). A de novo convergence of autism genetics and molecular neuroscience. *Trends Neurosci, 37*(2), 95-105. doi:10.1016/j.tins.2013.11.005

Krumm, N., Turner, T. N., Baker, C., Vives, L., Mohajeri, K., Witherspoon, K., . . . Eichler, E. E. (2015). Excess of rare, inherited truncating mutations in autism. *Nat Genet, 47*(6), 582-588. doi:10.1038/ng.3303

La Manno, G., Gyllborg, D., Codeluppi, S., Nishimura, K., Salto, C., Zeisel, A., . . . Linnarsson, S. (2016). Molecular Diversity of Midbrain Development in Mouse, Human, and Stem Cells. *Cell, 167*(2), 566-580.e519. doi:10.1016/j.cell.2016.09.027
10.1016/j.cell.2016.09.027.

La Manno, G., Soldatov, R., Zeisel, A., Braun, E., Hochgerner, H., Petukhov, V., . . . Kharchenko, P. V. (2018). RNA velocity of single cells. *Nature, 560*(7719), 494-498. doi:10.1038/s41586-018-0414-6

Lek, M., Karczewski, K. J., Minikel, E. V., Samocha, K. E., Banks, E., Fennell, T., . . . Exome Aggregation, C. (2016). Analysis of protein-coding genetic variation in 60,706 humans. *Nature, 536*(7616), 285-291. doi:10.1038/nature19057

Levy, J., Grotto, S., Mignot, C., Maruani, A., Delahaye-Duriez, A., Benzacken, B., . . . Tabet, A. C. (2018). NR4A2 haploinsufficiency is associated with intellectual disability and autism spectrum disorder. *Clin Genet, 94*(2), 264-268. doi:10.1111/cge.13383

Li, Y. E., Preissl, S., Hou, X., Zhang, Z., Zhang, K., Fang, R., . . . Ren, B. (2020). An Atlas of Gene Regulatory Elements in Adult Mouse Cerebrum. *bioRxiv*, 2020.2005.2010.087585. doi:10.1101/2020.05.10.087585

Lim, E. T., Uddin, M., De Rubeis, S., Chan, Y., Kamumbu, A. S., Zhang, X., . . . Walsh, C. A. (2017). Rates, distribution and implications of postzygotic mosaic mutations in autism spectrum disorder. *Nat Neurosci, 20*(9), 1217-1224. doi:10.1038/nn.4598

Lin, Y., Rajadhyaksha, A. M., Potash, J. B., & Han, S. (2018). A machine learning approach to predicting autism risk genes: Validation of known genes and discovery of new candidates. *bioRxiv*, 463547. doi:10.1101/463547

Louppe, G. (2014). Understanding random forests: From theory to practice. *arXiv preprint arXiv:1407.7502*.

Marianayagam, N. J., Sunde, M., & Matthews, J. M. (2004). The power of two: protein dimerization in biology. *Trends Biochem Sci, 29*(11), 618-625. doi:10.1016/j.tibs.2004.09.006

Martin, A., Calvigioni, D., Tzortzi, O., Fuzik, J., Warnberg, E., & Meletis, K. (2019). A Spatiomolecular Map of the Striatum. *Cell Rep, 29*(13), 4320-4333 e4325. doi:10.1016/j.celrep.2019.11.096

McLean, C. Y., Bristor, D., Hiller, M., Clarke, S. L., Schaar, B. T., Lowe, C. B., . . . Bejerano, G. (2010). GREAT improves functional interpretation of cis-regulatory regions. *Nat Biotechnol, 28*(5), 495-501. doi:10.1038/nbt.1630

McRae, J. F., Clayton, S., Fitzgerald, T. W., Kaplanis, J., Prigmore, E., Rajan, D., . . . Hurles, M. E. (2016). Prevalence, phenotype and architecture of developmental disorders caused by de novo mutation. *bioRxiv*. Retrieved from http://biorxiv.org/content/early/2016/04/22/049056.abstract

Miller, J. A., Ding, S. L., Sunkin, S. M., Smith, K. A., Ng, L., Szafer, A., . . . Lein, E. S. (2014). Transcriptional landscape of the prenatal human brain. *Nature, 508*(7495), 199-206. doi:10.1038/nature13185

Molyneaux, B. J., Arlotta, P., Menezes, J. R., & Macklis, J. D. (2007). Neuronal subtype specification in the cerebral cortex. *Nat Rev Neurosci, 8*(6), 427-437. doi:10.1038/nrn2151

Myers, S. M., Challman, T. D., Bernier, R., Bourgeron, T., Chung, W. K., Constantino, J. N., . . . Ledbetter, D. H. (2020). Insufficient Evidence for "Autism-Specific" Genes. *Am J Hum Genet, 106*(5), 587-595. doi:10.1016/j.ajhg.2020.04.004

Nguyen, H. T., Bryois, J., Kim, A., Dobbyn, A., Huckins, L. M., Munoz-Manchado, A. B., . . . Stahl, E. A. (2017). Integrated Bayesian analysis of rare exonic variants to identify risk genes for schizophrenia and neurodevelopmental disorders. *Genome Med, 9*(1), 114. doi:10.1186/s13073-017-0497-y

O'Roak, B. J., Vives, L., Girirajan, S., Karakoc, E., Krumm, N., Coe, B. P., . . . Eichler, E. E. (2012). Sporadic autism exomes reveal a highly interconnected protein network of de novo mutations. *Nature, 485*(7397), 246-250. doi:10.1038/nature10989

Ott, T., & Nieder, A. (2019). Dopamine and Cognitive Control in Prefrontal Cortex. *Trends Cogn Sci, 23*(3), 213-234. doi:10.1016/j.tics.2018.12.006

Parikshak, N. N., Luo, R., Zhang, A., Won, H., Lowe, J. K., Chandran, V., . . . Geschwind, D. H. (2013). Integrative functional genomic analyses implicate specific molecular pathways and circuits in autism. *Cell, 155*(5), 1008-1021. doi:10.1016/j.cell.2013.10.031

Petrovski, S., Wang, Q., Heinzen, E. L., Allen, A. S., & Goldstein, D. B. (2013). Genic intolerance to functional variation and the interpretation of personal genomes. *PLoS Genet, 9*(8), e1003709. doi:10.1371/journal.pgen.1003709

Pirooznia, M., Wang, T., Avramopoulos, D., Valle, D., Thomas, G., Huganir, R. L., . . . Zandi, P. P. (2012). SynaptomeDB: an ontology-based knowledgebase for synaptic genes. *Bioinformatics, 28*(6), 897-899. doi:10.1093/bioinformatics/bts040

Polioudakis, D., de la Torre-Ubieta, L., Langerman, J., Elkins, A. G., Shi, X., Stein, J. L., . . . Geschwind, D. H. (2019). A Single-Cell Transcriptomic Atlas of Human Neocortical Development during Mid-gestation. *Neuron, 103*(5), 785-801 e788. doi:10.1016/j.neuron.2019.06.011

Psych, E. C., Akbarian, S., Liu, C., Knowles, J. A., Vaccarino, F. M., Farnham, P. J., . . . Sestan, N. (2015). The PsychENCODE project. *Nat Neurosci, 18*(12), 1707-1712. doi:10.1038/nn.4156

Qi, H., Dong, C., Chung, W. K., Wang, K., & Shen, Y. (2016). Deep Genetic Connection Between Cancer and Developmental Disorders. *Human Mutation, 37*(10), 1042-1050. doi:10.1002/humu.23040

Ranganath, A., & Jacob, S. N. (2016). Doping the Mind: Dopaminergic Modulation of Prefrontal Cortical Cognition. *Neuroscientist, 22*(6), 593-603. doi:10.1177/1073858415602850

Reamon-Buettner, S. M., & Borlak, J. (2006). HEY2 mutations in malformed hearts. *Hum Mutat, 27*(1), 118. doi:10.1002/humu.9390

Regev, A., Teichmann, S. A., Lander, E. S., Amit, I., Benoist, C., Birney, E., . . . Human Cell Atlas Meeting, P. (2017). The Human Cell Atlas. *eLife, 6*, e27041. doi:10.7554/eLife.27041

Rice, A. M., & McLysaght, A. (2017). Dosage-sensitive genes in evolution and disease. *BMC Biol, 15*(1), 78. doi:10.1186/s12915-017-0418-y

Roadmap Epigenomics, C., Kundaje, A., Meuleman, W., Ernst, J., Bilenky, M., Yen, A., . . . Kellis, M. (2015). Integrative analysis of 111 reference human epigenomes. *Nature, 518*(7539), 317-330. doi:10.1038/nature14248

Ronemus, M., Iossifov, I., Levy, D., & Wigler, M. (2014). The role of de novo mutations in the genetics of autism spectrum disorders. *Nat Rev Genet, 15*(2), 133-141. doi:10.1038/nrg3585

Rosenberg, R. E., Law, J. K., Yenokyan, G., McGready, J., Kaufmann, W. E., & Law, P. A. (2009). Characteristics and concordance of autism spectrum disorders among 277 twin pairs. *Arch Pediatr Adolesc Med, 163*(10), 907-914. doi:10.1001/archpediatrics.2009.98

Rubenstein, J. L. (2011). Annual Research Review: Development of the cerebral cortex: implications for neurodevelopmental disorders. *J Child Psychol Psychiatry, 52*(4), 339-355. doi:10.1111/j.1469-7610.2010.02307.x

Ruzzo, E. K., Perez-Cano, L., Jung, J. Y., Wang, L. K., Kashef-Haghighi, D., Hartl, C., . . . Wall, D. P. (2019). Inherited and De Novo Genetic Risk for Autism Impacts Shared Networks. *Cell, 178*(4), 850-866 e826. doi:10.1016/j.cell.2019.07.015

Samocha, K. E., Robinson, E. B., Sanders, S. J., Stevens, C., Sabo, A., McGrath, L. M., . . . Daly, M. J. (2014). A framework for the interpretation of de novo mutation in human disease. *Nat Genet, 46*(9), 944-950. doi:10.1038/ng.3050

Sanyanusin, P., Schimmenti, L. A., McNoe, L. A., Ward, T. A., Pierpont, M. E., Sullivan, M. J., . . . Eccles, M. R. (1995). Mutation of the PAX2 gene in a family with optic nerve colobomas, renal anomalies and vesicoureteral reflux. *Nat Genet, 9*(4), 358-364. doi:10.1038/ng0495-358

Satterstrom, F. K., Kosmicki, J. A., Wang, J., Breen, M. S., De Rubeis, S., An, J. Y., . . . Buxbaum, J. D. (2020). Large-Scale Exome Sequencing Study Implicates Both Developmental and Functional Changes in the Neurobiology of Autism. *Cell, 180*(3), 568-584.e523. doi:10.1016/j.cell.2019.12.036

Shaikh, T. H., Gai, X., Perin, J. C., Glessner, J. T., Xie, H., Murphy, K., . . . Hakonarson, H. (2009). High-resolution mapping and analysis of copy number variations in the human genome: a data resource for clinical and research applications. *Genome Res, 19*(9), 1682-1690. doi:10.1101/gr.083501.108

Sifrim, A., Hitz, M. P., Wilsdon, A., Breckpot, J., Turki, S. H., Thienpont, B., . . . Hurles, M. E. (2016). Distinct genetic architectures for syndromic and nonsyndromic congenital heart defects identified by exome sequencing. *Nat Genet, 48*(9), 1060-1065. doi:10.1038/ng.3627

Song, M., Pebworth, M.-P., Yang, X., Abnousi, A., Fan, C., Wen, J., . . . Shen, Y. (2020). Cell-type-specific 3D epigenomes in the developing human cortex. *Nature*. doi:10.1038/s41586-020-2825-4

Steinberg, J., Honti, F., Meader, S., & Webber, C. (2015). Haploinsufficiency predictions without study bias. *Nucleic Acids Res, 43*(15), e101. doi:10.1093/nar/gkv474

Stoner, R., Chow, M. L., Boyle, M. P., Sunkin, S. M., Mouton, P. R., Roy, S., . . . Courchesne, E. (2014). Patches of disorganization in the neocortex of children with autism. *N Engl J Med, 370*(13), 1209-1219. doi:10.1056/NEJMoa1307491

Stricker, S. H., Koferle, A., & Beck, S. (2017). From profiles to function in epigenomics. *Nat Rev Genet, 18*(1), 51-66. doi:10.1038/nrg.2016.138

Stunnenberg, H. G., International Human Epigenome, C., & Hirst, M. (2016). The International Human Epigenome Consortium: A Blueprint for Scientific Collaboration and Discovery. *Cell, 167*(5), 1145-1149. doi:10.1016/j.cell.2016.11.007

Sun, Y. M., Wang, J., Qiu, X. B., Yuan, F., Li, R. G., Xu, Y. J., . . . Yang, Y. Q. (2016). A HAND2 Loss-of-Function Mutation Causes Familial Ventricular Septal Defect and Pulmonary Stenosis. *G3 (Bethesda), 6*(4), 987-992. doi:10.1534/g3.115.026518

Svensson, V., da Veiga Beltrame, E., & Pachter, L. (2019). A curated database reveals trends in single-cell transcriptomics. *bioRxiv*, 742304. doi:10.1101/742304

Takata, A., Miyake, N., Tsurusaki, Y., Fukai, R., Miyatake, S., Koshimizu, E., . . . Matsumoto, N. (2018). Integrative Analyses of De Novo Mutations Provide Deeper Biological Insights into Autism Spectrum Disorder. *Cell Rep, 22*(3), 734-747. doi:10.1016/j.celrep.2017.12.074

Taketani, T., Taki, T., Takita, J., Ono, R., Horikoshi, Y., Kaneko, Y., . . . Hayashi, Y. (2002). Mutation of the AML1/RUNX1 gene in a transient myeloproliferative disorder patient with Down syndrome. *Leukemia, 16*(9), 1866-1867. doi:10.1038/sj.leu.2402612

Trutzer, I. M., Garcia-Cabezas, M. A., & Zikopoulos, B. (2019). Postnatal development and maturation of layer 1 in the lateral prefrontal cortex and its disruption in autism. *Acta Neuropathol Commun, 7*(1), 40. doi:10.1186/s40478-019-0684-8

Turner, T. N., Hormozdiari, F., Duyzend, M. H., McClymont, S. A., Hook, P. W., Iossifov, I., . . . Eichler, E. E. (2016). Genome Sequencing of Autism-Affected Families Reveals Disruption of Putative Noncoding Regulatory DNA. *Am J Hum Genet, 98*(1), 58-74. doi:10.1016/j.ajhg.2015.11.023

Vastenhouw, N. L., & Schier, A. F. (2012). Bivalent histone modifications in early embryogenesis. *Curr Opin Cell Biol, 24*(3), 374-386. doi:10.1016/j.ceb.2012.03.009

Voineagu, I., Wang, X., Johnston, P., Lowe, J. K., Tian, Y., Horvath, S., . . . Geschwind, D. H. (2011). Transcriptomic analysis of autistic brain reveals convergent molecular pathology. *Nature, 474*(7351), 380-384. doi:10.1038/nature10110

Wagnon, J. L., Briese, M., Sun, W., Mahaffey, C. L., Curk, T., Rot, G., . . . Frankel, W. N. (2012). CELF4 regulates translation and local abundance of a vast set of mRNAs, including genes associated with regulation of synaptic function. *PLoS Genet, 8*(11), e1003067. doi:10.1371/journal.pgen.1003067

Wayne, S., Robertson, N. G., DeClau, F., Chen, N., Verhoeven, K., Prasad, S., . . . Smith, R. J. (2001). Mutations in the transcriptional activator EYA4 cause late-onset deafness at the DFNA10 locus. *Hum Mol Genet, 10*(3), 195-200. Retrieved from https://www.ncbi.nlm.nih.gov/pubmed/11159937

Willsey, A. J., Sanders, S. J., Li, M., Dong, S., Tebbenkamp, A. T., Muhle, R. A., . . . State, M. W. (2013). Coexpression networks implicate human midfetal deep cortical projection neurons in the pathogenesis of autism. *Cell, 155*(5), 997-1007. doi:10.1016/j.cell.2013.10.020

Wright, C. F., Fitzgerald, T. W., Jones, W. D., Clayton, S., McRae, J. F., van Kogelenberg, M., . . . study, D. D. D. (2015). Genetic diagnosis of developmental disorders in the DDD study: a scalable analysis of genome-wide research data. *Lancet, 385*(9975), 1305-1314. doi:10.1016/S0140-6736(14)61705-0

Wright, S. (1934). Physiological and Evolutionary Theories of Dominance. *The American Naturalist, 68*(714), 24-53. Retrieved from http://www.jstor.org/stable/2457086

Yuen, R. K. C., Merico, D., Bookman, M., Howe, J. L., Thiruvahindrapuram, B., Patel, R. V., . . . Scherer, S. W. (2017). Whole genome sequencing resource identifies 18 new candidate genes for autism spectrum disorder. *Nature Neuroscience, 20*(4), 602-+. doi:10.1038/nn.4524

Zaidi, S., Choi, M., Wakimoto, H., Ma, L., Jiang, J., Overton, J. D., . . . Lifton, R. P. (2013). De novo mutations in histone-modifying genes in congenital heart disease. *Nature, 498*(7453), 220-223. doi:10.1038/nature12141

Zhang, C., & Shen, Y. (2017). A Cell Type-Specific Expression Signature Predicts Haploinsufficient Autism-Susceptibility Genes. *Hum Mutat, 38*(2), 204-215. doi:10.1002/humu.23147

Zhang, M. J., Xia, F., & Zou, J. (2019). Fast and covariate-adaptive method amplifies detection power in large-scale multiple hypothesis testing. *Nat Commun, 10*(1), 3433. doi:10.1038/s41467-019-11247-0

Zhong, S., Zhang, S., Fan, X., Wu, Q., Yan, L., Dong, J., . . . Wang, X. (2018). A single-cell RNA-seq survey of the developmental landscape of the human prefrontal cortex. *Nature, 555*(7697), 524-528. doi:10.1038/nature25980
10.1038/nature25980. Epub 2018 Mar 14.

Zhou, V. W., Goren, A., & Bernstein, B. E. (2011). Charting histone modifications and the functional organization of mammalian genomes. *Nat Rev Genet, 12*(1), 7-18. doi:10.1038/nrg2905

Zhu, Y., Chen, Z., Zhang, K., Wang, M., Medovoy, D., Whitaker, J. W., . . . Wang, W. (2016). Constructing 3D interaction maps from 1D epigenomes. *Nat Commun, 7*, 10812. doi:10.1038/ncomms10812

Ziffra, R. S., Kim, C. N., Wilfert, A., Turner, T. N., Haeussler, M., Casella, A. M., . . . Nowakowski, T. J. (2020). Single cell epigenomic atlas of the developing human brain and organoids. *bioRxiv*, 2019.2012.2030.891549. doi:10.1101/2019.12.30.891549

Zikopoulos, B., & Barbas, H. (2013). Altered neural connectivity in excitatory and inhibitory cortical circuits in autism. *Front Hum Neurosci, 7*, 609. doi:10.3389/fnhum.2013.00609

Appendix

Supplementary table 2.1-2.14 can be found online:

https://www.nature.com/articles/s41467-018-04552-7

Supplementary table 3.1-3.6 can be found online:

https://www.biorxiv.org/content/10.1101/2020.06.15.153031v1.supplementary-material

www.ingramcontent.com/pod-product-compliance
Lightning Source LLC
LaVergne TN
LVHW041119150826
845673LV00007B/2129